Sourcebook for

Assessing & Maintaining Communication

Sourcebook for

Assessing & Maintaining Communication

Fiona Sugden-Best

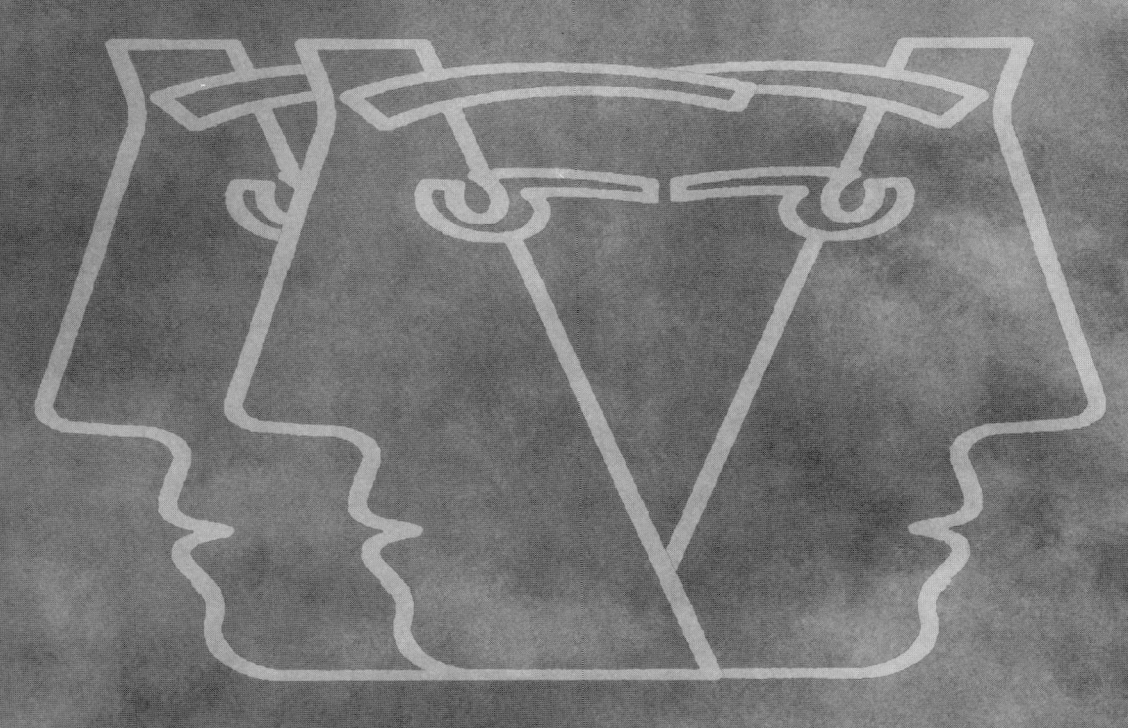

Speechmark

Speechmark Publishing Ltd
Telford Road • Bicester • Oxon OX26 4LQ • UK

First published in 2002 by
Speechmark Publishing Ltd, Telford Road, Bicester, Oxon, OX26 4LQ, UK

www.speechmark.net

002-4781/Printed in the United Kingdom/1010

British Library Cataloguing in Publication Data
Sugden-Best, Fiona
    Assessing and maintaining communication. - (Sourcebooks for neurodisability; 2)
    1. Language disorders – Treatment   2. Speech therapy
    I. Title
    616.8'55'06

ISBN 0 86388 305 2

Contents

Preface

The *Sourcebook for Assessing and Maintaining Communication* is a practical manual for those who work in a variety of clinical settings. In the course of my work with clients with moderate communication difficulties or clients needing support to maintain communication skills, both in a non-acute hospital setting and, most recently, in acute and intensive care settings, I have become increasingly aware of the paucity of suitable and readily available clinical material. Materials often have to be adapted, rewritten and redesigned to fulfil the needs of clients and carers alike.

This book has been written in response to this lack of provision and is designed for practising clinicians, whether experienced or newly qualified, and for students under clinical supervision. It includes a wealth of materials covering all aspects of therapy — and assessments including information sheets, programmes of breathing, oromotor and articulation exercises and alternative and augmentative communication forms and masters. These can be photocopied and used with clients and carers in different combinations, depending on the particular needs of the individual involved. Each chapter begins with a detailed description of the masters provided and suggestions regarding how these can best be used.

The assessments, stimulation and exercise sheets, firmly based on theory, have been extensively trialled with a range of client groups in acute, outpatient and domiciliary settings. As the contents are applicable to a wide range of clients, it is hoped that the book will become an invaluable and practical resource to clinicians working in a variety of settings.

Fiona Sugden-Best
2002

About the Author

Fiona Sugden-Best qualified as a speech and language therapist at City University, London, in 1988, where she returned to study for a MSc in Communication Disorders in 1993. She worked in a general position for Newham Health Authority before moving to the Royal Hospital for Neurodisability, where for seven-and-a-half years she managed a progressive neurological client group and provided cover on the rehabilitation wards, including the minimally responsive unit. She has also worked as Senior Speech & Language Therapist for Acute Neurosciences at The Royal London and Barts NHS Trust, and as Adult Team Co-ordinator for Redbridge Healthcare, covering a domiciliary caseload. She currently works as Head Speech & Language Therapist at The Children's Trust. She has always been actively involved in educating others, including speech and language therapists.

Acknowledgements

I would like to thank Jenny Sugden, my mother, who provided the original ideas for the illustrations; all the speech and language therapists where I have worked for the feedback they have given me; also Mark Sugden-Best, my husband, for all the times I said, 'But I've got to work on my book!'

Chapter 1

Oromotor Skills

This chapter includes handouts, information notes and record sheets relating to the following:

1 **An initial oromotor screen.** This should help the clinician decide which of the oromotor exercises later in the chapter may be of most use in improving or maintaining speech intelligibility. In the tongue section, sensory/visual prompting can be given by the use of fingers – for example, by touching the right corner of the client's mouth to indicate where the tongue needs to go.

2 **An assessment of oral movements.** This may be used with those clients for whom a basic oromotor screen is required. The clinician notes whether the client achieved the movement with verbal instruction, demonstration, written instruction, or a combination. This may prove useful in differentiating dysarthria from dyspraxia. The written instructions can be cut out and laminated, or covered in sticky-backed plastic.

3 **Speech exercising tips.** This sheet stresses the importance of being honest with your clinician.

4 **Facial exercises.** These exercises can be particularly useful to Parkinson's disease clients and others experiencing reduction in facial mobility, both unilaterally and bilaterally.

5 **Speech production.** This handout takes a basic look at the different types of speech sounds. It may be given out with any of the exercise sheets, including the breathing, intonation, pitch and resonance sheets found in Chapter 2, if considered useful to the client.

6 **Lip exercises.** This section contains an introductory sheet entitled 'Why do lip exercises?', as well as specific sets of exercises for improving or maintaining lip function with regard to range, rate and strength of movement. Specific techniques may be applied, such as icing, whereby the area of the face immediately above the muscle and/or supplied by the same cranial nerve is iced. Icing facilitates instantaneous effects, but these do not last, so exercises need to be done straight

away. Ice cubes, or alternatively crushed ice wrapped in a plastic or a surgical glove, may be used. Any wetness needs to be gently wiped away immediately. Slow brushing with ice is used to reduce spasticity – slow and rhythmic wiping or stroking with slight pressure, three times, along the line of the muscle with the tip of an ice cube. Fast icing is used to stimulate flaccid muscles; it involves rapid on/off flicking in the direction of the muscle movement, for up to five seconds. With both techniques it is important not to over ice, to prevent 'burns.'

Taptoment is light, rapid tapping with the finger ends – for example, over the orbicularis oris muscle, to stimulate blood supply to the muscle and increase sensation. This technique should be applied alternately to the strong and weak side immediately prior to, for example, lip rounding.

These techniques are also useful for the facial exercises. Strength exercises should be used with caution with progressive disorders that result in increased fatigue.

7 **Tongue exercises.** This section includes an introductory sheet entitled 'Why do tongue exercises?' and sets of exercises that focus on improving or maintaining the range, rate and strength of tongue movement. Again, strength exercises should be used with caution with progressive disorders.

8 **Jaw exercises.** These are for use with clients with reduction in jaw mobility.

9 **Soft palate exercises.** This section includes a basic description of soft palate movement, and is intended for clients with disordered nasal resonance.

10 **Drooling techniques.** These give clients basic techniques to help lessen this difficulty.

11 **Record sheets.** These are provided for each of the exercise programmes, divided into daily recording units over a three-week period. If the client is not going to be seen for more than three weeks, then additional record sheets can be given. It is important to highlight the honesty policy in the exercising tips.

Initial Oromotor Screen

Name _____ Date _____

Diagnosis _____

Key:
Reduction   *Increase*
↓ (mild)   ↓↓ (moderate)   ↓↓↓ (severe)   + (mild)   ++ (moderate)   +++ (severe)

Score according to whether the movement was demonstrated, carried out in response to a verbal command, or a combination of the two. Do each movement three times to note for fatigue.

Facial expression						
Movement	**Demonstration**		**Verbal command**		**Demonstration and verbal command**	
	right	left	right	left	right	left
Raise eyebrows (*Frontalis*)						
Frown (*Corrugator Supercilii*)						
Screw up eyes tightly (*Orbicularis Oculi*)						
Scrunch up nose (*Procerus*)						
Smile (*Zygomaticus Major*)						
Protrude upper lips to show gums (*Levator Labii Superioris*)						
Draw down lips and tense neck (*Depressor Labii Inferioris & Platysma*)						
Purse lips (as in whistling) (*Orbicularis Oris*)						
Pout bottom lip (*Mentalis*)						
Draw down sides of mouth (*Depressor Anguli Oris*)						

Comments

Initial Oromotor Screen ...continued

Key:
Reduction   *Increase*
↓ (mild)   ↓↓ (moderate)   ↓↓↓ (severe)   + (mild)   ++ (moderate)   +++ (severe)
D – Demonstrated   V – Verbal command   V+D – Both demonstrated/Verbal command

Lips

Movement	Symmetry	Range	Strength	Rate/speed
At rest				
Lips together				
Round 'oo'				
Open wide 'ah'				
Spreading 'ee'				
Alternating 'ah/oo'				
Alternating 'oo/ee'				
Alternating 'ah/oo/ee'				
Puff cheeks				
Close left side only				
Close right side only				
'mm/bb/ww/rr'				

Tongue

Movement	Symmetry	Range	Strength	Rate/time
At rest				
Protrusion				
Side-to-side				
Elevation				
Depression				
Rotate around lips				
Rotate inside lips				
Push tip into cheek				
'dd/nn'				
'gg'				
'd/g'				

Palate

Movement	Symmetry	Range	Strength	Rate/time
At rest				
'ah' 'ah'				

Initial Oromotor Screen ...continued

Comments

Lips

Tongue

Palate

AUTOMATIC SPEECH

1 Count 1 to 10   1 2 3 4 5 6 7 8 9 10   /10

2 Days of the week   Sunday Monday Tuesday Wednesday
Thursday Friday Saturday   /7

3 Months of the year   January February March April May
June July August September October
November December   /12

4 Address   (score 5 for total accuracy to 0 for no response)   /5

REPETITION

1 Sound   B __ K __ L __ D __ P __ M __ T __   /7

2 Word
Dog _____
Clock _____
Banana _____
Caterpillar _____
Sensible _____
Persevere _____
Festivity _____   /7

3 Sentence
The car is blue. _____
Keep cleaning the kitchen. _____
The cap is green. _____
Danny dislikes dates. _____
Take time for tea. _____   /5

Initial Oromotor Screen ...continued

Scores for automatic/repetition tasks

Speech task	Sub-section	Score
Automatic speech	Count to 10	/10
	Days of the week	/7
	Months of the year	/12
	Address	/5
	Total	/34
Repetition	Sound	/7
	Word	/7
	Sentence	/5
	Total	/19

Comments and conclusions

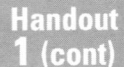

Assessment of Oral Movement

Name _____

Date Programme Commenced _____

Oral movement	Verbal instruction	Demonstration	Written instruction
Smile			
Open your mouth wide			
Round your lips			
Press your lips firmly together			
Puff out your cheeks			
Bite your lower lip			
Bite your upper lip			
Show me your teeth			
Click your teeth together			
Stick out your tongue			
Point your tongue to your nose			
Point your tongue to your chin			
Move your tongue from side to side			
Raise your tongue tip behind your top teeth			
Raise the back of your tongue			

Key P = Present   A = Absent   G = Groping   D = Different movement made   N/A = Not assessed

Written Instructions for Assessment of Oral Movement

Smile.

Open your mouth wide.

Round your lips.

Press your lips firmly together.

Puff out your cheeks.

Bite your lower lip.

Bite your upper lip.

Show me your teeth.

Click your teeth together.

Stick out your tongue.

Point your tongue to your nose.

Point your tongue to your chin.

Move your tongue from side to side.

Raise your tongue tip behind your top teeth.

Raise the back of your tongue.

Speech Exercising Tips

Name _____ Date _____

1 Don't do your exercises when you are tired.

2 Don't be afraid to ask if you are unsure about the correct way to do any of the exercises on the following sheets.

3 Try to enjoy doing your exercises. Think about the positive benefits of doing them regularly; otherwise, you will find any excuse to keep leaving them until later.

4 Try to practise the exercises for short periods of time on a regular basis.

5 Find regular times that fit in easily with your normal daily routine.

6 If there is a genuine reason to miss out on exercising, for example, you were unwell/or were away for the weekend with friends, don't worry. If you try to fit them in when there is not enough time available you will probably not do them properly.

7 When asked in therapy sessions, don't pretend to have done your exercises when you have not. Otherwise it will be impossible to determine if the current programme is the most appropriate and works for you as an individual.

8 Sit wherever is most comfortable for you. Start with your face relaxed and mouth closed. If possible, have a mirror handy so that you can see your face in it.

9 Try to do the exercises in private, or with someone you know well, so you don't feel too self-conscious.

Facial Exercises

Name _____ Date _____

Facial expression is an important way for us to communicate information to others non-verbally. It tells them a lot about our personality. It is important, therefore, to keep our facial muscles well exercised.

Do each movement three times, relaxing between movements. Do these exercises in front of a mirror if you can. Notice any asymmetry in your face – that is, one side moving more than the other.

1 Raise your eyebrows, wrinkling your forehead. Then let your eyebrows slowly descend. Check the furrows have disappeared before repeating.

2 Frown.

3 Open your eyes wide.

4 Close your eyes tightly, wrinkling your nose at the same time. Then slowly release the tension.

5 Wrinkle your nose.

6 Yawn.

7 Make an exaggerated smile.

8 Round or pout your lips.

9 Press your lips together tightly. Feel your cheeks tightening. Release the tension.

10 Clench your teeth together tightly. Feel how tense your jaw is. Now relax slowly. Open your lips and let your jaw rest in an easy, relaxed position.

11 Practise making different facial expressions indicating the following:

Surprise	Anger
Fear	Pain
Happiness	Confusion
Sadness	Concern

Ask someone to guess which emotion you are depicting by your facial expression.

Speech Production

Name _____ Date _____

The different speech sounds you produce are made by your lips, tongue, teeth, palate, vocal cords and air coming up from your lungs.

Production of each individual speech sound is very complex, and this complexity increases when individual sounds are strung together to form words.

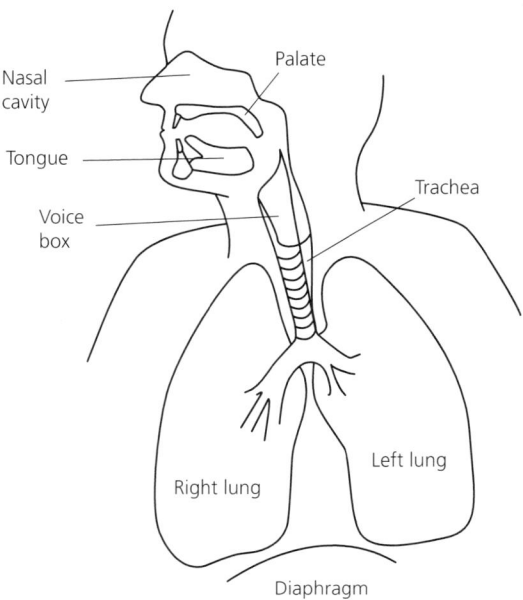

There are a number of different types of speech sounds:

1 **Voiced sounds** occur when the vocal cords vibrate – for example, 'b' and 'g.' You should be able to feel a humming sensation as your larynx (voicebox) vibrates.

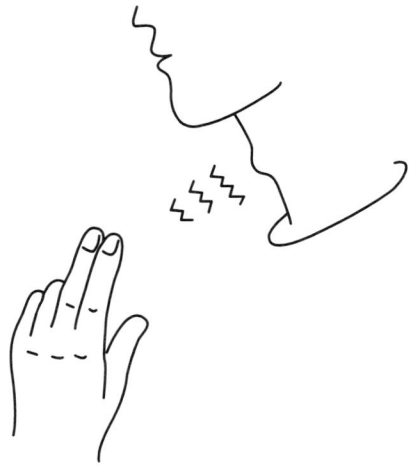

Speech Production ...*continued*

Voiceless sounds occur when your vocal cords do not vibrate – for example, 'p' and 'k', where no vibration should be felt at your larynx.

2 **Nasal sounds** occur when your palate is lowered to allow air to travel down your nose – for example, 'm' and 'n'. If you hold a metal spoon under your nose, you should see it cloud from the hot air escaping down your nostrils.

Non-nasal sounds occur when your palate is raised. This shuts off the nasal cavity and you will not see the spoon clouding – for example, 'f' and 'p'.

3 **Lip sounds** occur when your lips are involved in articulating the sound in some way:

◆ Firm contact – for example, 'p' and 'b'

◆ Contact with the upper teeth – for example, 'f' and 'v'

◆ Closed lip rounding – for example, 'w' and 'r'

◆ Open lip rounding – for example, 'ah'

◆ Spreading – for example, 'ee'.

4 **Tongue tip sounds** occur when the tip of your tongue presses behind your top front teeth – for example, 't' and 'n'.

5 **Tongue back sounds** occur when the back of your tongue is raised towards your palate – for example, 'k' and 'g'.

6 A **plosive** is a sound you produce that explodes on being said, because your speech organs are firmly together – for example, 'p' and 'g'.

7 A **fricative** is a sound you produce when two speech organs are brought very close together, forcing the air through the resulting narrowing and making a friction noise – for example, 's' and 'th'.

You have been given the following set of exercises as you appear to have difficulty in articulating your sounds clearly. These exercises are specifically tailored to help you improve the intelligibility of your speech.

Why do Lip Exercises?

Name _____ Date _____

Good range, rate and strength of lip movements are important for you to produce clearly articulated speech.

These movements include rounding, spreading, opening and closing:

◆ Speech sounds requiring good lip closure are: 'b', 'p' and 'm'.

◆ Speech sounds requiring good lip rounding are: 'r' and 'w'.

◆ For all the other speech sounds, your lips adopt various degrees of openness.

The exercises have been selected to help you achieve better range and/or rate and/or strength of lip movements.

Many of the exercises need to be repeated several times in order for you to gain full benefit from them. This will mean that your muscles become used to repetition and do not become tired. In normal conversational speech your muscles move extremely quickly.

Using a mirror will help you to see how well you are managing to accomplish each exercise.

Lip Exercises for Range of Movement

Name _____ Date _____

Do each exercise three times, relaxing between movements.

1 Open your mouth as wide as you can.
Relax.

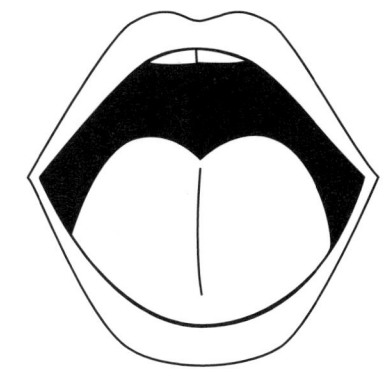

2 Raise your top lip only to show your
top teeth/gums.
Relax.

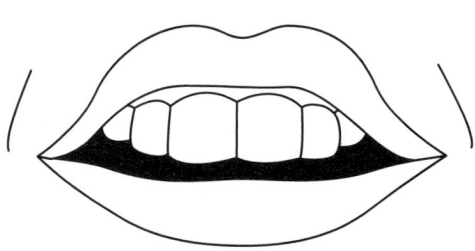

3 Lower your bottom lip only to show your bottom
teeth/gums.
Relax.

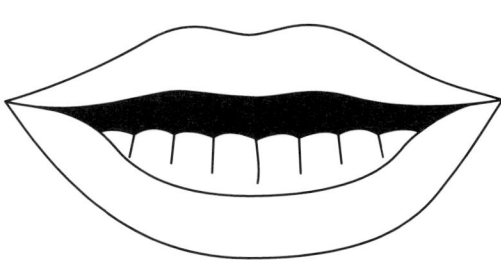

4 Press your lips
firmly together
and hum.
Relax.

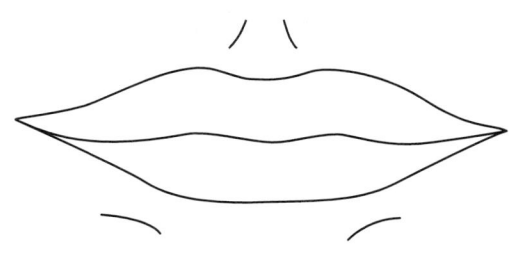

5 Stretch your lips
into an 'ee' shape/
exaggerated smile.
Relax.

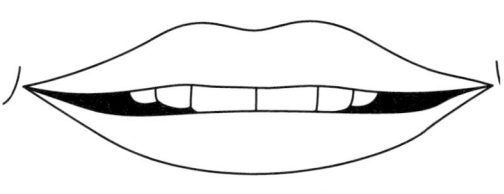

6 Round your lips
into an 'oo' shape/
shape to whistle.
Relax.

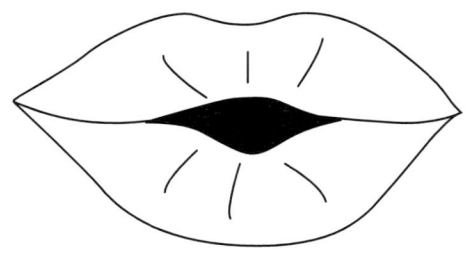

7 Hold the left corner of your
mouth together.
Relax.

Hold the right corner of your
mouth together.
Relax.

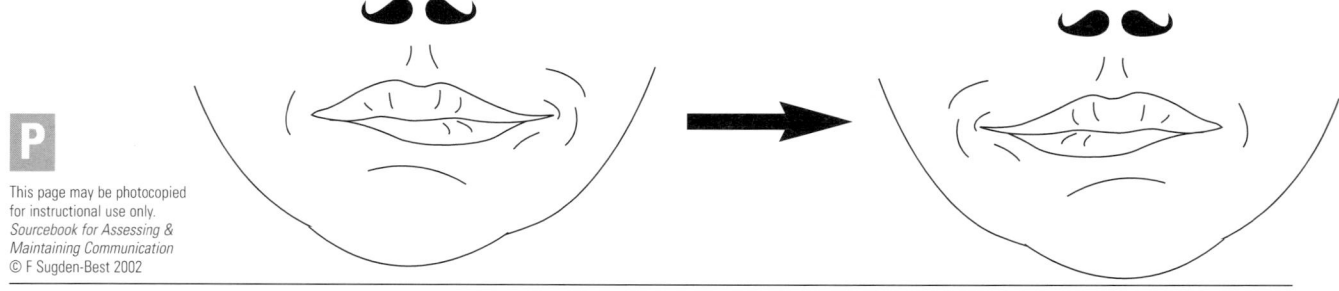

Lip Exercises for Rate of Movement

Name _____ Date _____

Do each exercise three times, relaxing between movements.

1 Round your lips into an 'oo' shape as in 'boot' and then spread them into an 'ee' shape as in 'feet', making the movements as slowly and smoothly as possible.

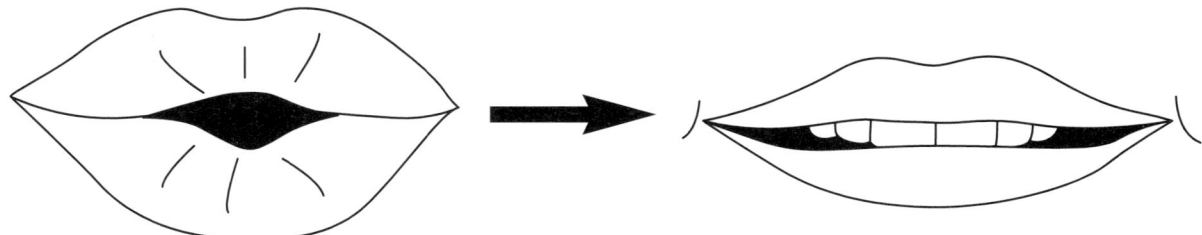

Now repeat the movement as quickly and precisely as possible.

2 Open your mouth into a wide 'ah' shape as when yawning, and then round to an 'oo' shape. Make the movements as slowly and smoothly as possible.

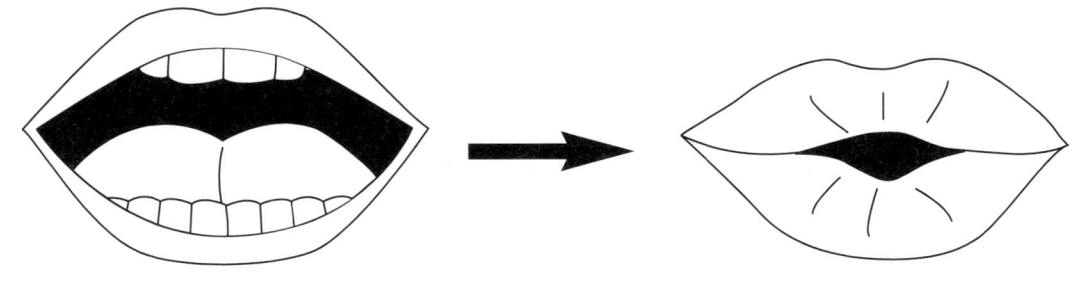

Now repeat the movement as quickly and precisely as possible.

3 Make the three movements 'ah' to 'oo' to 'ee', as slowly and smoothly as possible.

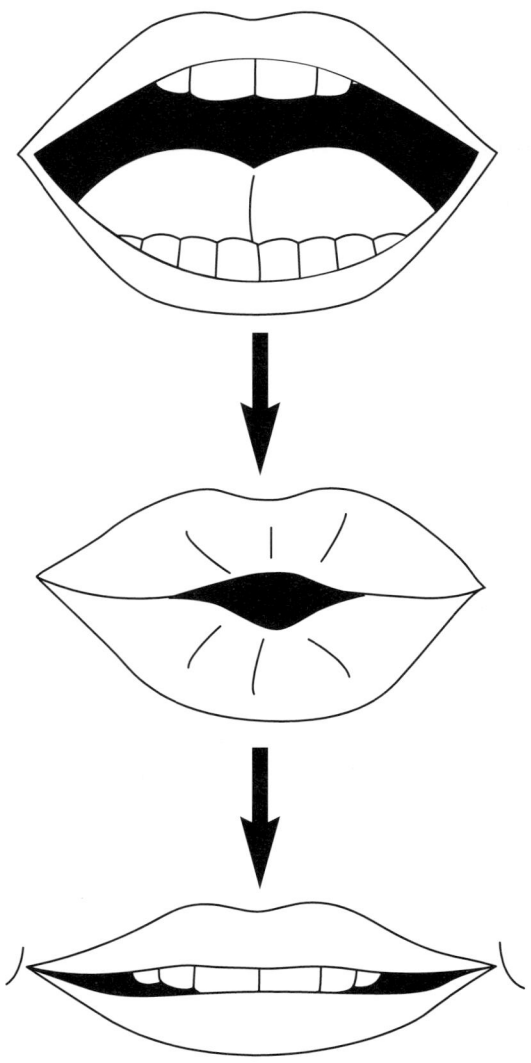

Now repeat the movement as quickly and precisely as possible.

4 Press your lips firmly together while saying a clear 'b' sound.

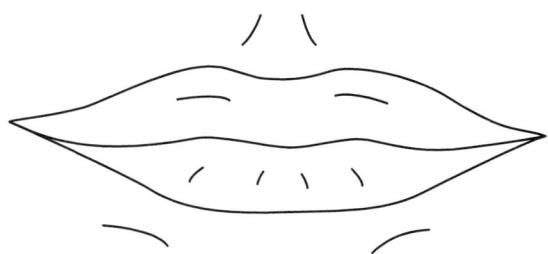

Now repeat several clear 'b's at an increased rate.

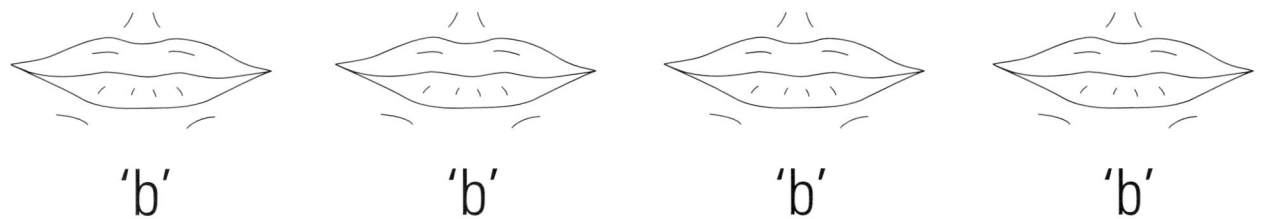

'b'   'b'   'b'   'b'

Repeat again using the sounds 'p' and 'm'.

5 Hold the left corner only of your mouth together, and then hold the right corner of your mouth together. Move between the two movements as quickly but as precisely as possible.

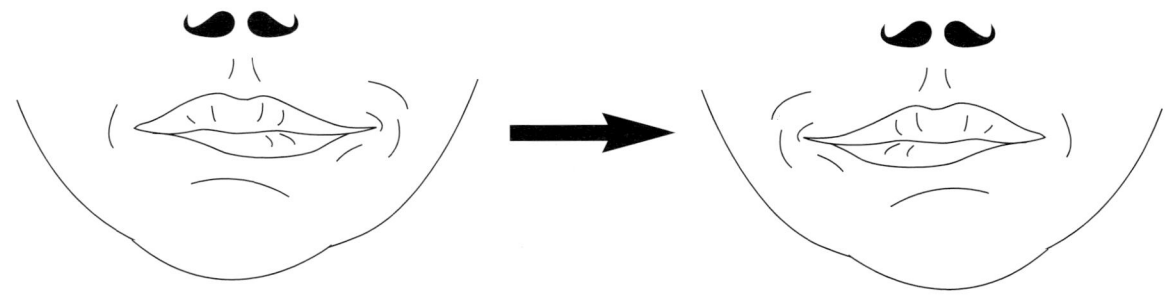

Lip Exercises for Strength of Movement

Name _____ Date _____

Do each exercise three times, relaxing between movements.

1 Press your lips together as firmly as you can.

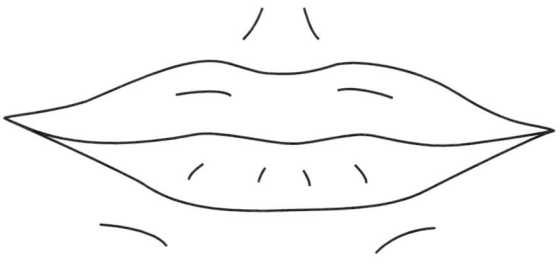

Hold for 10 seconds.

2 Place a spatula between your lips, in the centre, and firmly press your lips together (not using your teeth). Hold it for 10 seconds.

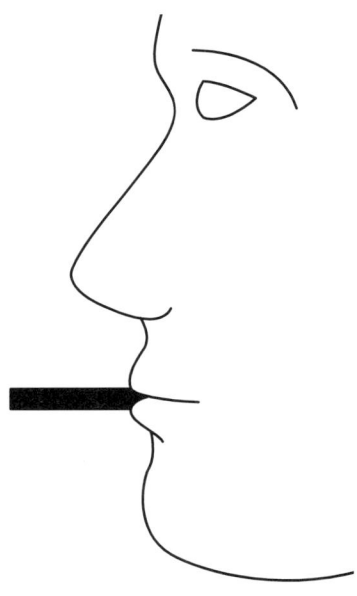

3 Tap a finger on the free end of the spatula, and do not allow it to fall out of your mouth. Try balancing a small coin on the end, or try to pull the spatula from your lips.

4 Try holding the spatula to the right side of your lips; then to the left. Again press with your finger/put coin on the end.

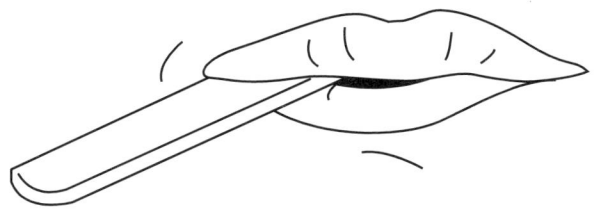 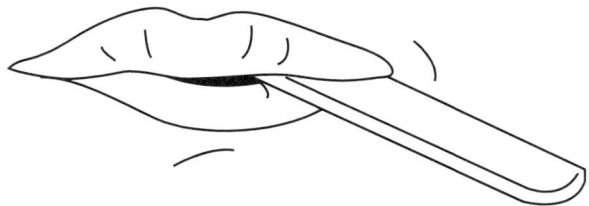

5 Press your lips firmly together and puff up your cheeks with air. Check whether both sides look even. Continue to breathe in and out of your nose. Hold for 10 seconds.

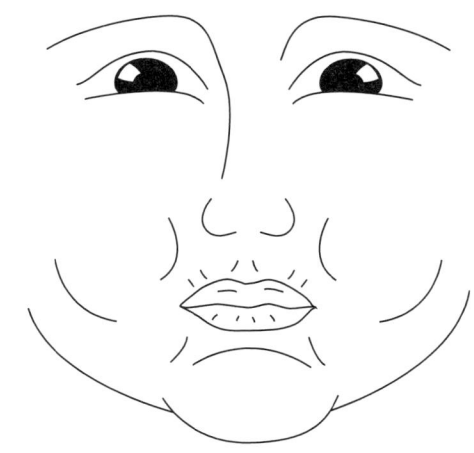

6 Try pushing, or get someone else to push, against your inflated cheeks. Remember to keep your lips firmly together.

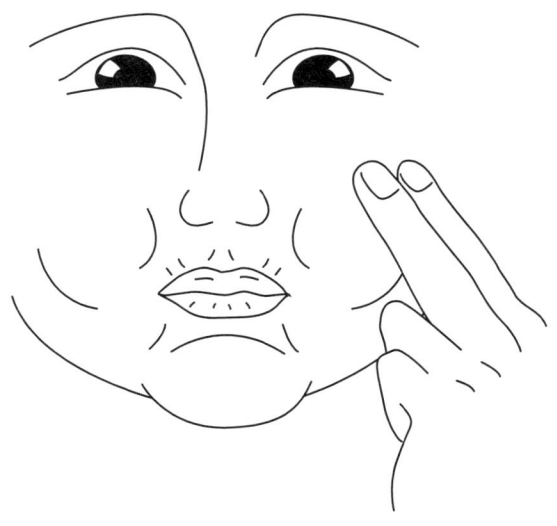

7 Try to puff up just your right cheek. Hold for five seconds. Then just your left cheek. Hold for five seconds.

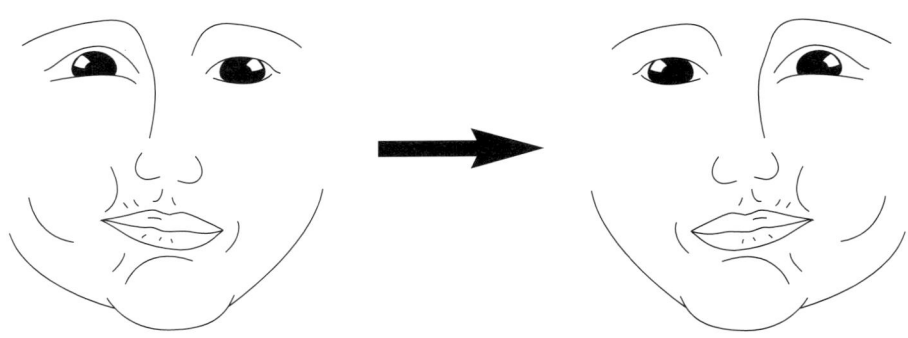

8 Hold your lips together using your index finger above and second finger below. Try to open your mouth, while at the same time trying to close it with your fingers.

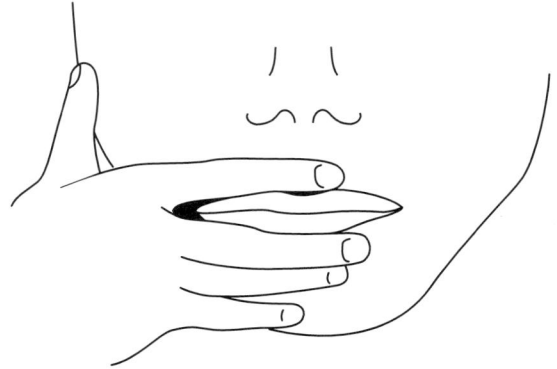

9 Round your lips into a tight 'oo' shape. Hold for five seconds.

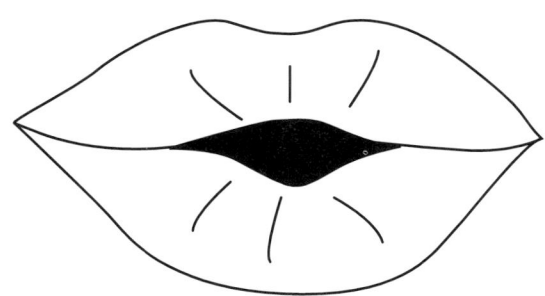

10 Try placing your lips tightly around a straw. Blow out while trying to keep your cheeks puffed up with air.

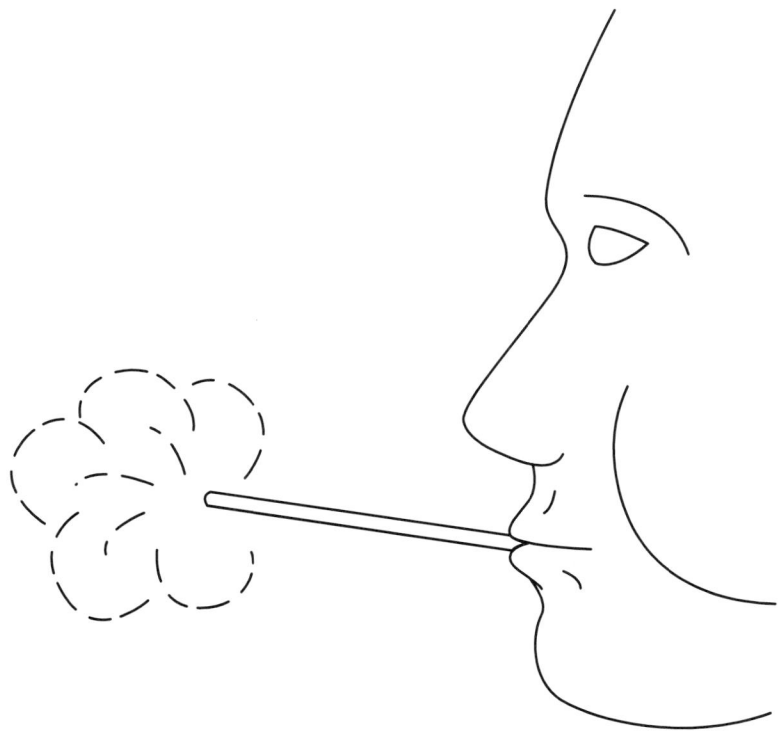

Why do Tongue Exercises?

Name _____ Date _____

Good range, rate and strength of tongue movements are important for the production of clearly articulated speech.

These movements include poking out, pulling back, side to side and circular movements of the tongue.

◆ Speech sounds that require the tip of the tongue to be raised are 't','d','l' and 'n'.

◆ Speech sounds requiring some tongue tip control are 'th', 's', 'z' and 'ch'.

◆ Speech sounds that require the back of the tongue to be raised are 'k', 'g' and 'ing'.

The attached exercises have been selected to help achieve better range and/or rate and/or strength of tongue movements.

Many of the exercises need to be repeated several times to gain full benefit, so that the muscles become used to repetition and do not become tired. In normal conversational speech the muscles move extremely quickly.

Using a mirror will help you to see how well you are managing to accomplish each exercise.

Tongue Exercises for Range of Movement

Name _____ Date _____

Do each exercise three times, relaxing between movements.

1 Stick out your tongue as far as possible. Make sure it is straight and not resting on your lips. It may help to have someone hold up a finger for you to touch with your tongue. Then pull it back in.

2 Using the tip of your tongue, lick across your top lip from the right to the left corner. Do this as slowly as possible.

Repeat the exercise going from the left to the right corner.

3 Using the tip of your tongue, lick across your bottom lip from right to left as slowly as possible.

Repeat this exercise going from left to right.

4 Stick out your tongue and try to touch your nose with the tip of your tongue.

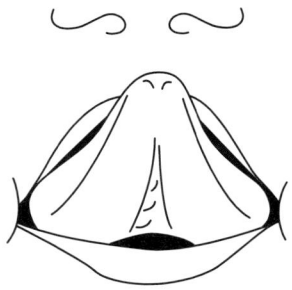

5 Stick out your tongue and try to reach as far down your chin as possible with the tip of your tongue.

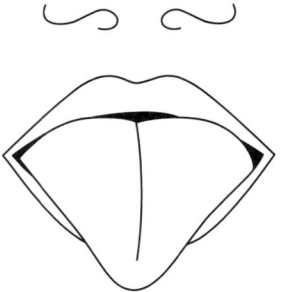

6 Combine exercises 4 and 5 moving your tongue up and down without drawing it back into your mouth.

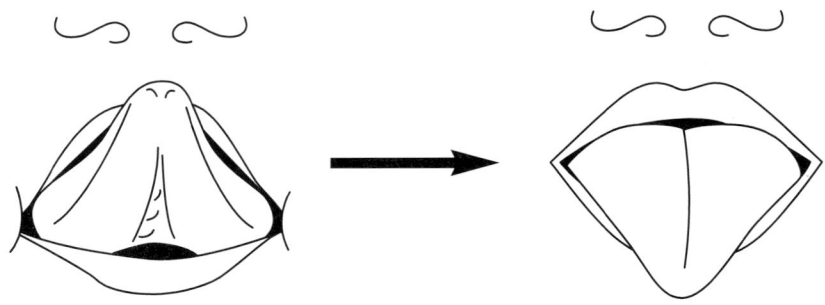

7 With the tip of your tongue touch the right corner of your lip, and then the left corner, on the outside.

8 With your tongue tip, move from nose to chin, then from right to left.

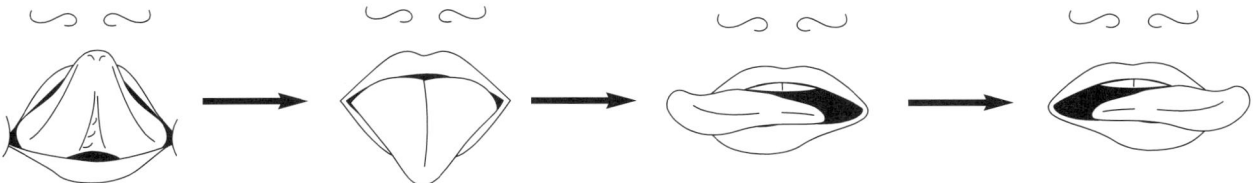

9 Raise your tongue tip inside your mouth, in front of your top teeth.

Repeat the exercise, lowering your tongue tip in front of your bottom teeth.

10 With your tongue tip, lick in front of your top teeth, from right to left, at the level of the gum.

Repeat the exercise going from left to right.

11 With your tongue tip, lick in front of your bottom teeth, from right to left, at the level of the gum.

Repeat the exercise from left to right.

12 Raise your tongue tip to touch just behind your top teeth, as if saying the sound 'd'.

Touch further back.

Touch further back again.

13 Repeat exercise 12 with your mouth open.

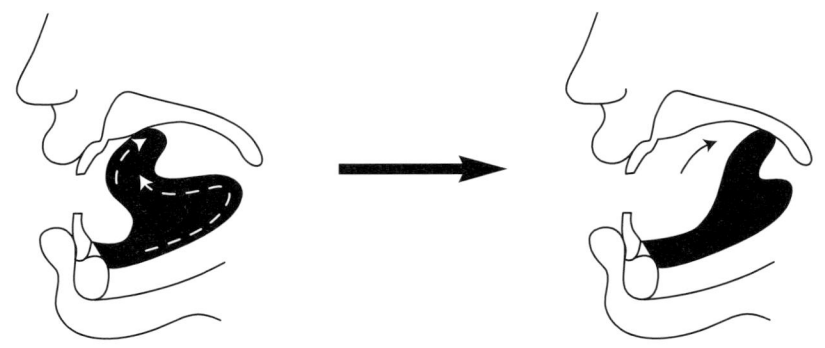

14 With your tongue tip, lick behind your top teeth from right to left, at the level of the gum.

Repeat the exercise going from left to right.

15 With your tongue tip, lick behind your bottom teeth from right to left at the level of the gum.

Repeat the exercise going from left to right.

16 Try to push out your right cheek using your tongue tip.

Repeat for the left cheek.

17 Try to raise the back of your tongue against the roof of your mouth, as if saying the sound 'g'.

18 Repeat exercise 17 with your mouth open.

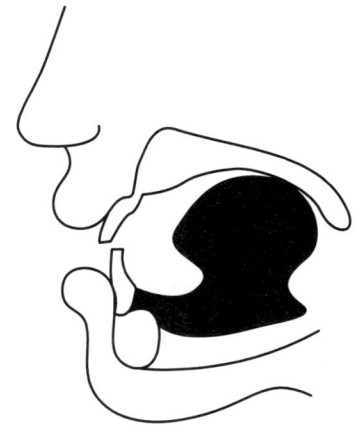

Tongue Exercises for Rate of Movement

Name _____ Date _____

Do each exercise three times, relaxing between movements.

1 Stick your tongue as far out of your mouth as you can, and then pull it back in again.

Repeat the movement as quickly and smoothly as possible.

2 With your tongue outside your mouth, point your tongue tip up towards your nose, and then point it down towards your chin.

Repeat the movement as quickly and smoothly as possible.

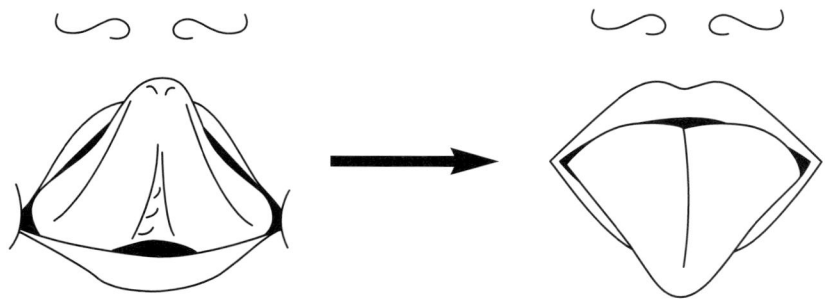

3 With your tongue outside your mouth, first point your tongue tip to the right-hand corner of your mouth, and then to the left.

Repeat the movement as quickly and smoothly as possible.

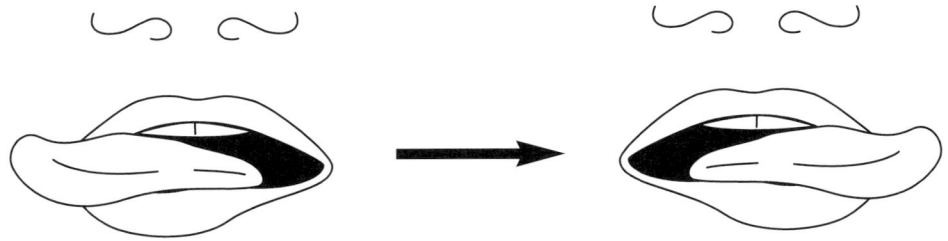

Repeat going from left to right.

4 Press your tongue tip behind your top teeth inside your mouth.

Say five 'd' sounds as quickly but as clearly as possible.

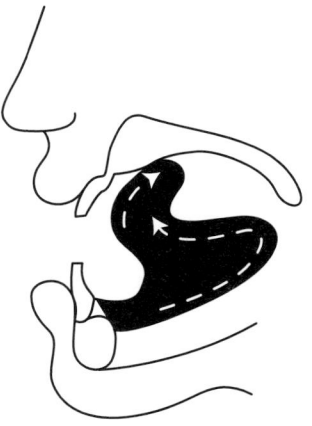

5 Press the back of your tongue up to the top of your mouth.

Say five 'g' sounds as quickly but as clearly as possible.

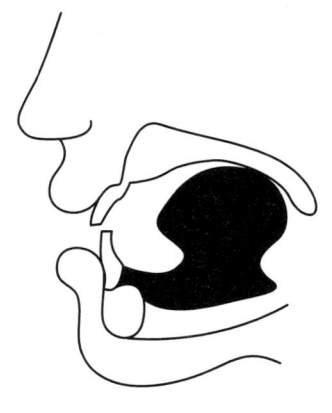

6 Move from 'd' to 'g' as quickly but as precisely as possible, and then from 'g' to 'd'.

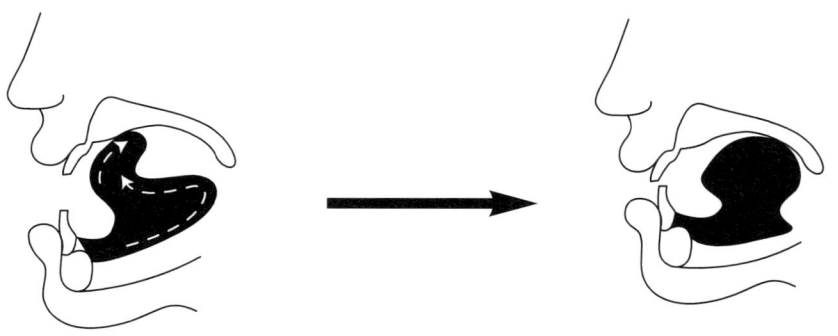

7 Push your tongue tip into your right cheek and then into your left cheek. Repeat as quickly as possible.

Repeat, moving from left to right cheek.

Tongue Exercises for Strength of Movement

Name _____ Date _____

Do each exercise three times, resting between movements. You may need a friend/ partner to help you with these exercises.

1 Hold a finger, teaspoon, spatula or toothbrush in front of your lips and touch it with the tip of your tongue pressing as firmly as you can.

    Using your tongue, try to push the object away.

2 Holding the object to the right-hand corner of your mouth, point your tongue tip outside and touch it as firmly as you can. Repeat to the left.

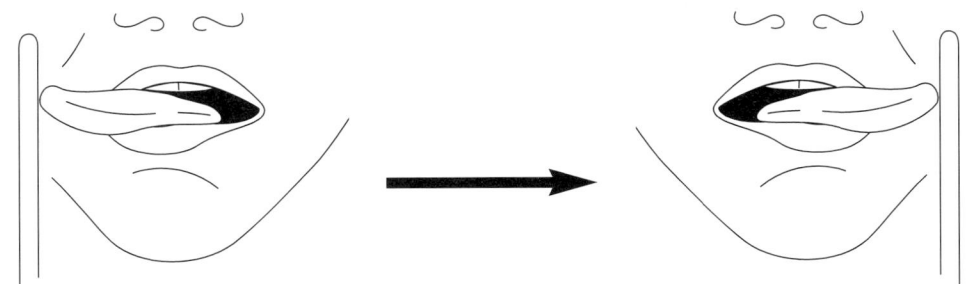

Still using your tongue, try to push the object away.

3 Stick out your tongue just past your bottom lip. Place a spatula, finger, toothbrush or teaspoon under your extended tongue, and press down firmly on it. Push up with the object, resisting the pressure.

4 Stick out your tongue, this time with the spatula, finger, toothbrush or teaspoon above your tongue. Press firmly against it. Push down with the object, resisting the pressure.

5 Press your tongue tip as firmly as you can behind your top teeth inside your mouth, as when saying the sound 'd'.

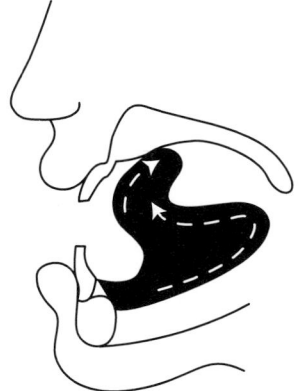

Then press firmly against your lower teeth.

6 Press the back of your tongue as firmly as you can against the roof of your mouth, as when saying the sound 'g'.

7 Place your hand on your right cheek and push your tongue hard against it inside; then repeat on the left side.

Jaw Exercises

Name _____ Date _____

The lowering and raising of your jaw is important for well-articulated speech. The following exercises are designed to aid good jaw movement.

Do each exercise five times, resting between movements. You may need a friend/partner to help you with some of the exercises.

1 Lower your jaw as far as you are able, by opening your mouth wide, and then close it again.

You can gradually increase jaw opening by using a stack of spatulas. Increase the number in the stack. Slide them in on one side of the mouth, through to the

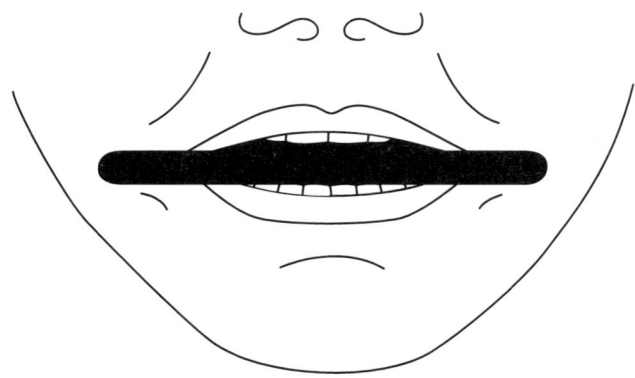

other side – for example, Day 1 = two spatulas, Day 2 = three spatulas, etc. Keep them in position for a few seconds.

2 Drop your jaw gently and move it slowly to the right and then to the left.

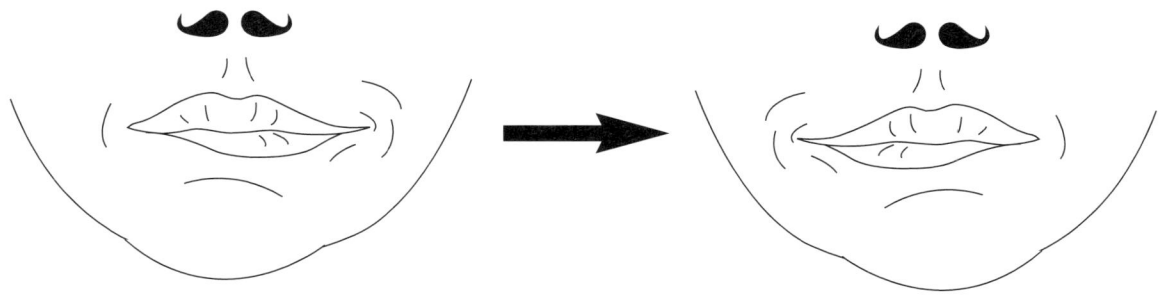

Repeat the exercise moving from left to right.

3 Drop your jaw gently and make exaggerated chewing movements with your mouth closed.

Repeat the exercise with your mouth open.

4 Place a hand or fist under your jaw/chin and as you try to keep your jaw open, push upwards.

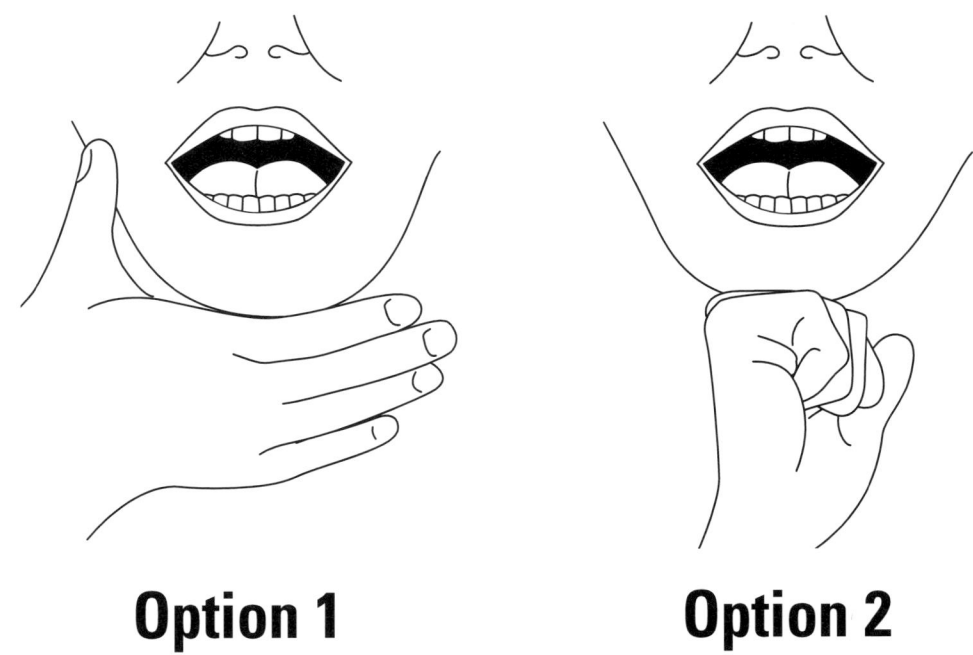

Option 1   **Option 2**

5 Place a fist under your jaw/chin firmly as you try to open your mouth.

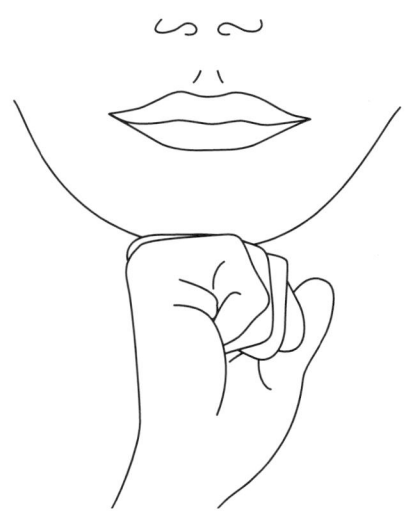

Why do Soft Palate Exercises?

Name _____ Date _____

The soft palate is in the roof of the mouth at the back. When it is **raised**, air is unable to pass down the nose, resulting in non-nasal sounds – for example, 't', 'd', 'k' and 'g'.

Now, try snorting down your nose and feel the airflow. When the palate is **lowered**, air passes out through your nose as well as out of your mouth, making nasal sounds – that is, 'n','m' and 'ng'.

If the soft palate is not working properly, the non-nasal sounds can become nasal, and vice versa.

The following exercises are designed to help your palate to work more effectively. Do each exercise five to 10 times, three times a day.

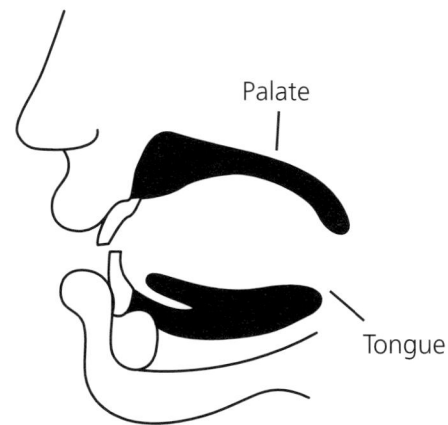

Soft Palate Exercises

Name _____ Date _____

Do each exercise five times, resting between movements.

1 Yawn.

2 Puff out your cheeks with air. Continue to breathe in and out of your nose.

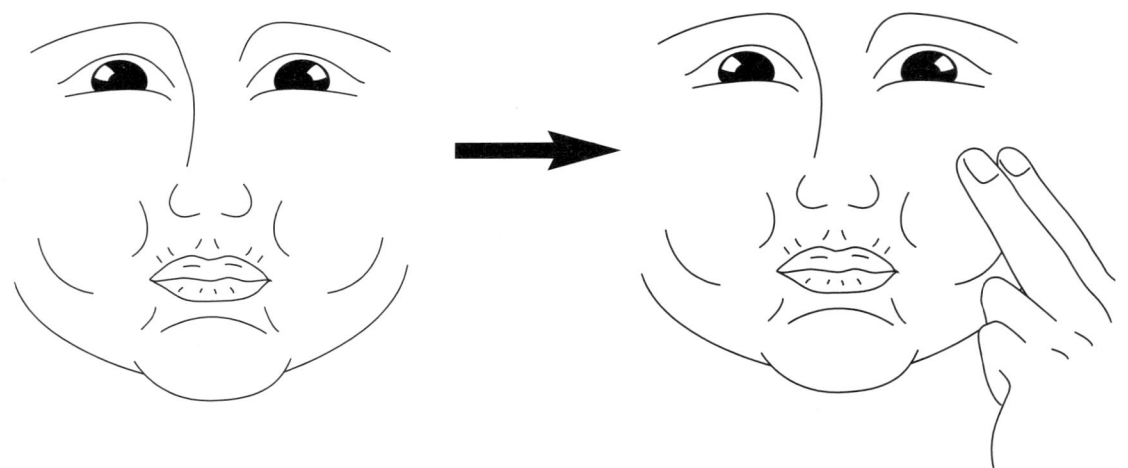

Try yourself, or get someone else, to press a finger against your inflated cheeks. Remember to keep your lips firmly together.

Do not allow the air to escape through your mouth or nose.
Hold for 10 seconds.

3 Try to puff up your right cheek. Hold for five seconds.

Puff up your left cheek. Hold for five seconds.

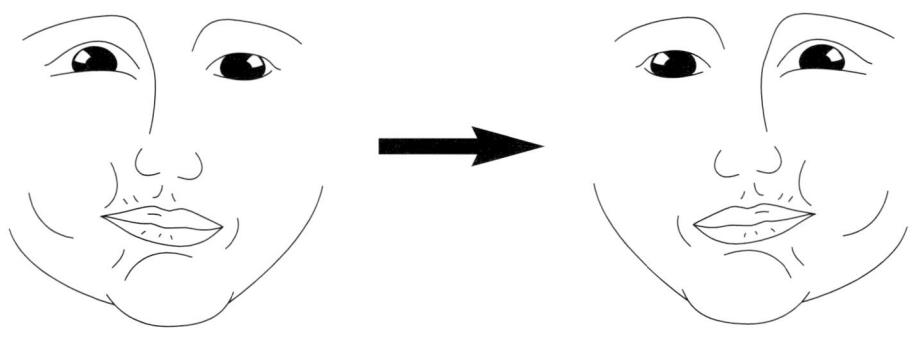

4 Blow out through a straw.

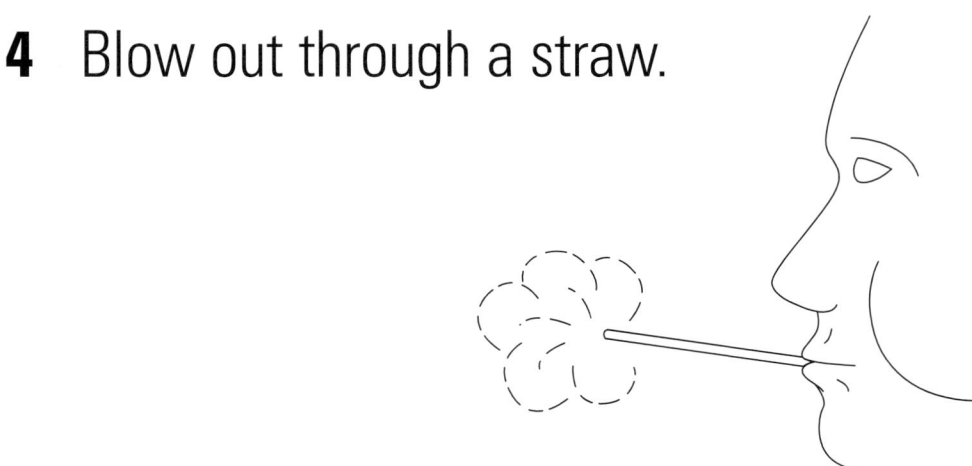

5 Blow out through a straw with your finger, or someone else's, over the end. Keep the air in the straw for five to 10 seconds.

6 Suck a small amount of liquid up through a straw and transfer it to another container, without losing any.

7 For this exercise it is important that the order of the sequence of movements is maintained.

- ◆ Hum, keeping the lips together
- ◆ Stop humming
- ◆ Puff out your cheeks with air
- ◆ Say 'p' as you release the air through your lips.

8 Practise saying 'ssss' without allowing any air to come out through your nose.

9 Make five 'ah' sounds. Pause between each 'ah'.

10 Make the following sounds, pausing in between:

a. . . . . .p   a. . . . . .p   a. . . . . .p

a. . . . . . . .b   a. . . . . . . .b   a. . . . . . . .b

a. . . . . . . .m   a. . . . . . . .m   a. . . . . . . .m

a. . . . . . . .n   a. . . . . . . .n   a. . . . . . . .n

Gradually put the two sounds together, with no pause between.

11 Make the following sounds, pausing in between:

ma......pa   ma......pa   ma......pa

ma......ba   ma......ba   ma......ba

na......ta   na......ta   na......ta

na......da   na......da   na......da

ka......ing   ka......ing   ka......ing

ga......ing   ga......ing   ga......ing

Gradually put the two sounds together, with no pause between.

12 Make the following sounds, pausing in between:

m......ba   m......ba   m......ba

n......da   n......da   n......da

n......ga   n......ga   n......ga

Gradually put the two sounds together, with no pause between.

Tips to Alleviate Dribbling

Name _____ Date _____

Due to weakness of your lips on either one or both sides, you are experiencing problems with dribbling. The following are suggestions to reduce or eliminate the problem. You may also have been given a specific set of exercises to help strengthen the lip muscles.

1 Try to keep your mouth closed at all times, and breathe in and out through your nose.

2 Get into the habit of swallowing at regular intervals, even if you feel there is no need, to keep your mouth free of excess saliva.

3 As soon as you feel some saliva escape from your mouth, try to push it back in with your tongue tip, or pull it back in with your top lip.

4 Try to reduce your use of tissues, as this can result in soreness and dry skin around the mouth area.

Name _____

Date Programme Commenced _____

FACIAL EXERCISES

DAYS	Monday			Tuesday			Wednesday			Thursday			Friday			Saturday			Sunday		
WEEKS	1	2	3	1	2	3	1	2	3	1	2	3	1	2	3	1	2	3	1	2	3
Raise eyebrows																					
Frown																					
Eyes wide open																					
Eyes tight shut																					
Wrinkle nose																					
Yawn																					
Exaggerated smile																					
Round/pout lips																					
Lips firmly together																					
Clench teeth together																					
Facial expressions																					

Tick when you do each exercise each day over the next three weeks. If you do the exercise more than once, then represent this by the number of ticks in the box.

Record Sheet

Name _____

Date Programme Commenced _____

LIP EXERCISES FOR RANGE OF MOVEMENT

DAYS	Monday			Tuesday			Wednesday			Thursday			Friday			Saturday			Sunday		
WEEKS	1	2	3	1	2	3	1	2	3	1	2	3	1	2	3	1	2	3	1	2	3
Open mouth wide																					
Show top teeth																					
Show bottom teeth																					
Lips firm together																					
'ee' shape																					
'oo' shape																					
Left corner/right corner																					

Tick when you do each exercise each day over the next three weeks. If you do the exercise more than once, then represent this by the number of ticks in the box.

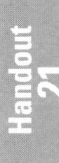

Record Sheet

Name _____

Date Programme Commenced _____

LIP EXERCISES FOR RATE OF MOVEMENT

DAYS	Monday			Tuesday			Wednesday			Thursday			Friday			Saturday			Sunday		
WEEKS	1	2	3	1	2	3	1	2	3	1	2	3	1	2	3	1	2	3	1	2	3
'oo' to 'ee'																					
'ah' to 'oo'																					
'ah' to 'oo' to 'ee'																					
Lips firm together and 'b'																					
Left corner to right corner																					

Tick when you do each exercise each day over the next three weeks. If you do the exercise more than once, then represent this by the number of ticks in the box.

Record Sheet

Name _____

Date Programme Commenced _____

LIP EXERCISES FOR STRENGTH OF MOVEMENT

DAYS	Monday			Tuesday			Wednesday			Thursday			Friday			Saturday			Sunday		
WEEKS	1	2	3	1	2	3	1	2	3	1	2	3	1	2	3	1	2	3	1	2	3
Press lips firm together (10 seconds)																					
Spatula between lips (10 seconds)																					
Tap spatula with finger/balance coins/pull spatula from lips																					
Spatula in right side																					
Spatula in left side																					
Puff up cheeks (10 seconds)																					

Record Sheet

Name _____

Date Programme Commenced _____

LIP EXERCISES FOR STRENGTH OF MOVEMENT

DAYS	Monday			Tuesday			Wednesday			Thursday			Friday			Saturday			Sunday		
WEEKS	1	2	3	1	2	3	1	2	3	1	2	3	1	2	3	1	2	3	1	2	3
Puff up right cheek (5 seconds)																					
Puff up left cheek (5 seconds)																					
Lips together, use fingers to resist opening																					
Round lips/'oo' shape (5 seconds)																					
Place lips tight around a straw																					

Tick when you do each exercise each day over the next three weeks. If you do the exercise more than once, then represent this by the number of ticks in the box.

Record Sheet

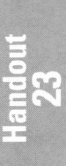

Name _____ Date Programme Commenced _____

TONGUE EXERCISES FOR RANGE OF MOVEMENT

DAYS	Monday			Tuesday			Wednesday			Thursday			Friday			Saturday			Sunday		
WEEKS	1	2	3	1	2	3	1	2	3	1	2	3	1	2	3	1	2	3	1	2	3
Stick tongue far out																					
Tongue tip licking top lip																					
Tongue tip licking bottom lip																					
Tongue tip to nose																					
Tongue tip to chin																					
Tongue tip to nose to chin																					
Tongue tip to right corner																					
Tongue tip to left corner																					
Tongue tip to nose to chin to left to right																					
Tongue tip licking in front of top teeth																					

Record Sheet

Name _____   Date Programme Commenced _____

TONGUE EXERCISES FOR RANGE OF MOVEMENT

DAYS	Monday			Tuesday			Wednesday			Thursday			Friday			Saturday			Sunday		
WEEKS	1	2	3	1	2	3	1	2	3	1	2	3	1	2	3	1	2	3	1	2	3
Tongue tip licking in front of bottom teeth																					
Tongue tip behind top teeth/'d' (mouth closed)																					
Tongue tip behind top teeth/'d' (mouth open)																					
Tongue tip licking behind top teeth																					
Tongue tip licking behind bottom teeth																					
Tongue tip into right cheek																					
Tongue tip into left cheek																					
Raise back of tongue/'g' (mouth closed)																					
Raise back of tongue/'g' (mouth open)																					

Tick when you do each exercise each day over the next three weeks. If you do the exercise more than once, then represent this by the number of ticks in the box.

Record Sheet

Name _____ Date Programme Commenced _____

TONGUE EXERCISES FOR RATE OF MOVEMENT

DAYS	Monday			Tuesday			Wednesday			Thursday			Friday			Saturday			Sunday		
WEEKS	1	2	3	1	2	3	1	2	3	1	2	3	1	2	3	1	2	3	1	2	3
Stick tongue in and out																					
Tongue tip to nose to chin																					
Tongue tip from right to left corner																					
Tongue tip from left to right corner																					
Tongue tip behind top teeth/'dddd'																					

Record Sheet

Name _____ Date Programme Commenced _____

TONGUE EXERCISES FOR RATE OF MOVEMENT

DAYS	Monday			Tuesday			Wednesday			Thursday			Friday			Saturday			Sunday		
WEEKS	1	2	3	1	2	3	1	2	3	1	2	3	1	2	3	1	2	3	1	2	3
Tongue back to top of mouth/'gggg'																					
Say 'd' to 'g'																					
Tongue tip inside from right to left cheek																					
Tongue tip inside from left to right cheek																					

Tick when you do each exercise each day over the next three weeks. If you do the exercise more than once, then represent this by the number of ticks in the box.

Record Sheet

Name _____

Date Programme Commenced _____

TONGUE EXERCISES FOR STRENGTH OF MOVEMENT

DAYS	Monday			Tuesday			Wednesday			Thursday			Friday			Saturday			Sunday		
WEEKS	1	2	3	1	2	3	1	2	3	1	2	3	1	2	3	1	2	3	1	2	3
Press tongue tip on spatula																					
Push tongue tip with spatula, resist pressure																					
Press tongue tip to spatula right corner																					
Tongue to spatula right corner, resist pressure																					
Press tongue tip to spatula left corner																					
Tongue to spatula left corner, resist pressure																					
Tongue tip down on spatula																					

Record Sheet

Name _____

Date Programme Commenced _____

TONGUE EXERCISES FOR STRENGTH OF MOVEMENT

DAYS	Monday			Tuesday			Wednesday			Thursday			Friday			Saturday			Sunday		
WEEKS	1	2	3	1	2	3	1	2	3	1	2	3	1	2	3	1	2	3	1	2	3
Tongue tip down on spatula, resist pressure																					
Tongue tip with spatula above																					
Tongue tip with spatula above, resist pressure																					
Press tongue tip firmly behind top teeth/'d'																					
Press tongue tip firmly to lower teeth																					
Press tongue back firmly to top of mouth/'g'																					
Press tongue tip hard in to right cheek/left cheek																					

Tick when you do each exercise each day over the next three weeks. If you do the exercise more than once, then represent this by the number of ticks in the box.

Record Sheet

Name _____ Date Programme Commenced _____

JAW EXERCISES

DAYS	Monday			Tuesday			Wednesday			Thursday			Friday			Saturday			Sunday		
WEEKS	1	2	3	1	2	3	1	2	3	1	2	3	1	2	3	1	2	3	1	2	3
Open jaw wide																					
Move jaw to right																					
Move jaw to left																					
Exaggerated chewing movements (mouth open)																					
Exaggerated chewing movements (mouth closed)																					
Hand to jaw resist to keep open (option 1)																					
Fist to jaw resist to keep open (option 2)																					
Fist to jaw, try to open mouth																					

Tick when you do each exercise each day over the next three weeks. If you do the exercise more than once, then represent this by the number of ticks in the box.

Record Sheet

Name _____ Date Programme Commenced _____

SOFT PALATE EXERCISES

DAYS	Monday			Tuesday			Wednesday			Thursday			Friday			Saturday			Sunday		
WEEKS	1	2	3	1	2	3	1	2	3	1	2	3	1	2	3	1	2	3	1	2	3
Puff cheeks with air																					
Press cheeks with finger																					
Puff up right cheek (5 seconds)																					
Puff up left cheek (5 seconds)																					
Blow out through straw																					
Hold air in straw with finger on end																					
Suck liquid into straw and transfer																					

Name _____

Date Programme Commenced _____

SOFT PALATE EXERCISES

DAYS	Monday			Tuesday			Wednesday			Thursday			Friday			Saturday			Sunday		
WEEKS	1	2	3	1	2	3	1	2	3	1	2	3	1	2	3	1	2	3	1	2	3
Firm lips to hum to puff up to release on 'p'																					
'sssss'																					
'ah' 5 times																					
Exercise 10																					
Exercise 11																					
Exercise 12																					

Tick when you do each exercise each day over the next three weeks. If you do the exercise more than once, then represent this by the number of ticks in the box.

Chapter 2

Voice Parameters, Questionnaires and Breathing

This chapter includes handouts, questionnaires and information sheets relating to the following:

1   **Client questionnaire.** This gives the clinician a clear picture of what the client feels about their communication and whether they consider the current therapeutic intervention to have been beneficial.

2   **'How well do I communicate?'** This questionnaire gives the clinician an idea of how the client views their communication skills.

3   **'How do you rate your speech?'** This is a useful sheet to introduce in the first session, to give a baseline rating for both clinician and client.

4   **Personal communication history form.** This is for the client to fill in, prior to attending the initial session. It is especially useful for giving background information to assistants and volunteers who are following a work programme devised by the speech and language therapist. It helps to identify functional situations and areas of specific interest to focus on.

5   **Relaxation exercises.** 'Why relax?' is an introductory sheet giving information for all client groups regarding the importance of relaxation for communication. 'Are you a relaxed person?' is a questionnaire that directs the clinician towards contributing factors that may result in the person being stressed. There is also a set of relaxation exercises for the whole body, neck, shoulders and arms.

6   **Posture.** 'Why is posture important for speech and voice production?' is a general information sheet for the client to take away.

7   **Breath control and voice.** This section comprises an information sheet and a set of exercises to promote breathing, voice production and breath control. 'Let's breathe' is a useful sheet for voice and dysarthric clients alike. This is a useful section to accompany the oromotor exercise sheets as an overall maintenance package with progressive clients.

8 Pitch. This section includes a number of exercises with accompanying diagrams that visually represent pitch changes, diminuendo and crescendo. These can be used with clients experiencing specific problems with pitch control. Use of auditory feedback – that is tape recording – is especially helpful when working on this area as well as proprioceptive feedback – that is, feeling laryngeal movement with the hands as the pitch changes and describing the 'feeling' inside. The diagrams can be photocopied and filled with black or hatched patterns, or coloured in with a variety of bright colours for clearer visual representation. Coloured samples are provided in the appendixes.

9 Intonation. This section includes a set of exercises with some visual representation of direction of stress patterns. Again, tape recording may prove beneficial.

10 Resonance. This section comprises an information sheet and set of exercises for improving resonance.

With all the exercise sheets, it is important for the clinician to indicate to the client whether all or some of the exercises should be carried out on a regular basis. Factors such as fatigability and over-exertion on the part of the client need to be taken into account.

Client Questionnaire

Name _____ Date _____

Therapy attended (circled   *Dysphasia*   *Dysarthria*   *Dysphonia*   *AAC*
by therapist if applicable):   Group   Individual

1   My current speech difficulties are:

_____

_____

_____

2   I communicate as much as I would like to with *(tick all appropriate boxes)*:
    ☐ Nursing staff   ☐ Family   ☐ New people
    ☐ Therapists   ☐ Friends   ☐ Other residents

3   I feel I am understood by *(mark N (Never), O (Occasionally), U (Usually) or A (Always))*:
    ___ Nursing staff   ___ Family   ___ New people
    ___ Therapists   ___ Friends   ___ Other residents

4   I communicate most regularly with *(mark 1 to 6, with 1 for the people you
communicate with most and 6 for those you communicate with least)*:
    ___ Nursing staff   ___ Family   ___ New people
    ___ Therapists   ___ Friends   ___ Other residents

5   I am able to make myself understood *(tick the correct response)*:
    ☐ Never   ☐ Occasionally   ☐ Usually   ☐ Always

6   I feel I am generally able to communicate *(tick all appropriate boxes)*:
    ☐ Basic needs, eg, *hungry*   ☐ Personal information
    ☐ Small talk/general chit chat   ☐ Feelings
    ☐ Serious conversation

7   Which of the above are difficult to communicate?

Why?

Client Questionnaire ...*continued*

8 Topics I avoid communicating about are:

_____

_____

_____

Why?

_____

_____

9 I try to make myself understood by:

_____

_____

_____

10 I know people have understood me because:

_____

_____

_____

11 I like help in making myself understood?   ☐ YES ☐ NO
If yes, what kind of help is most useful?

_____

_____

_____

Is there anything you do not like people to do?

_____

_____

_____

12 When I am not understood I feel *(tick all appropriate boxes)*:
☐ Responsible ☐ Anxious ☐ Guilty ☐ Impatient ☐ Frustrated ☐ Angry
Anything else?

_____

_____

13 I give up without communicating my message *(tick all appropriate boxes)*:
☐ Never   ☐ Occasionally   ☐ Usually   ☐ Always

Client Questionnaire ...continued

14 When people do not understand me, I respond by:

_____

_____

15 When people have not understood me, I want them to:

_____

_____

16 I know people have not understood me when they:

_____

_____

17 I initiate communication with *(mark N (Never), O (Occasionally), U (Usually) or A (Always))*:

__ Nursing staff   __ Family   __ New people

__ Therapists   __ Friends   __ Other residents

Fill in the following questions if you have had therapy.

18 Do you feel the speech and language sessions you have had so far have been beneficial?   ☐ YES ☐ NO
Why?

19 Do you feel you could benefit from further sessions?   ☐ YES ☐ NO
Why?

20 Do you feel there is anything else/different that would be helpful in sessions?

Thank you for taking the time to fill out this questionnaire.

How Well do I Communicate?

Name _____ Date _____

Tick the response that you feel relates most appropriately to your communication abilities.

1 I have difficulty communicating with other people.

Strongly disagree ☐ Disagree ☐ Agree ☐ Strongly agree ☐

2 I understand why I am having difficulties communicating with others.

Strongly disagree ☐ Disagree ☐ Agree ☐ Strongly agree ☐

3 I often become frustrated when communicating with other people.

Strongly disagree ☐ Disagree ☐ Agree ☐ Strongly agree ☐

4 I often choose to say nothing, rather than communicate.

Strongly disagree ☐ Disagree ☐ Agree ☐ Strongly agree ☐

5 I communicate with my friends and family as much as I did before.

Strongly disagree ☐ Disagree ☐ Agree ☐ Strongly agree ☐

6 I have changed the way I communicate with others.

Strongly disagree ☐ Disagree ☐ Agree ☐ Strongly agree ☐

7 My lifestyle has had to change to accommodate my communication difficulties.

Strongly disagree ☐ Disagree ☐ Agree ☐ Strongly agree ☐

8 I use other ways to communicate with others, not just by talking.

Strongly disagree ☐ Disagree ☐ Agree ☐ Strongly agree ☐

How Do You Rate Your Speech?

Name _____ Date _____

Tick the boxes that refer to your voice. Score at the start of therapy, half-way through
and at the end of the initial block.

(++ means too much of a given parameter)

Speech Parameter			Scores			Dates
Volume	++ quiet 1	2	3	4	++ loud 5	
Speed	++ slow 1	2	3	4	++ fast 5	
Pitch	++ deep 1	2	3	4	++ high 5	
Clarity	++ slurred 1	2	3	4	++ clear 5	
How clear do you feel your speech is to others?	++ poor 1	2	3	4	++ good 5	
How much does your speech worry you?	all the time 1	2	3	4	it doesn't 5	
Overall speech rating	++ poor 1	2	3	4	++ good 5	

(Note: Your clinician will discuss with you as to whether they would agree with your
scores).

Personal Communication History Form

Name _____ Date _____

The following information will be helpful when we are treating your communication difficulty. The more we know about you, your family, friends and interests, the easier it is for us to tailor the sessions to your needs. If you are unable to write clearly, please ask someone who knows you well to help you fill in the form.

1   Personal details

Name/Nickname _____ DOB _____

Address _____

Phone no _____

GP's name and address _____

_____

If you are not the client, what relationship do you have to them? *(eg, wife, son, nurse)*

Who lives with you? *(eg, wife, live alone, live in a residential home, live in a nursing home, etc.)*

Do you wear glasses for reading?   ☐ Yes ☐ No

(If so, would you please make sure that you bring them to therapy sessions.)

Do you have a history of hearing problems?   ☐ Yes ☐ No

(If you wear a hearing aid, would you please make sure that you wear it or bring it to therapy sessions.)

Do you wear dentures?   Yes ☐   No ☐

                                               Top ☐   Bottom ☐

Do you wear them all the time?   ☐ Yes ☐ No

What is/was your job? *(Please give as much detail as possible and mention previous jobs.)*

Personal Communication History Form ...continued

Prior to your illness, were you a good speller? ☐ Yes ☐ No

Are you retired? ☐ Yes ☐ No

Were you in the Armed Services? ☐ Yes ☐ No

(If so, please give details.)

_____

_____

_____

2 Social details

Family

Include the names/nicknames of anybody seen by you on a regular basis.

Name of wife/husband:

Name of son	Wife's name	Grandchildren's names & ages	Where do they live?
1			
2			
3			

Name of daughter	Husband's name	Grandchildren's names & ages	Where do they live?
1			
2			
3			

Names of close relatives (brothers, sisters, in-laws, etc) and any relevant details. (List only those you are likely to mention regularly.)

1
2
3
4
5
6

Personal Communication History Form ...continued

Friends
Include the names/nicknames with any relevant details (*eg, workmate, neighbour, etc*). Tick any who are seen regularly.

1

2

3

4

Has anything happened to any of the named family members and friends recently that might be on your mind (*eg, wedding, death, passed an exam*)?

_____

_____

Pets
Give the names and types of pets belonging to your family.

_____

_____

3 Hobbies and interests

Hobbies
Do you have any hobbies (*eg, knitting, gardening, films*)? Give details.

_____

_____

Places
Are there any places of particular interest to you (*eg, holiday haunts, weekend visits*)?

_____

_____

Travel
Have you ever been abroad?   ☐ Yes ☐ No
(If so, give details.)

_____

_____

Have you ever lived anywhere else for a period of time?   ☐ Yes ☐ No
(If so, give details.)

_____

_____

Personal Communication History Form ...continued

Topics to avoid
Can you think of any topics that ought to be avoided, because of their
painful association for you?

_____

_____

_____

Sport
Are there any any sports, teams, etc that you are interested in?

_____

_____

_____

Did you play any sport before your illness?

_____

_____

Clubs/Societies
Name any clubs or societies that you belong to.

_____

_____

_____

Religion
Are you affiliated to any religious organisations?
(eg, Church, Temple, Mosque)? (If so, give details.)　　☐ Yes ☐ No

_____

_____

_____

Television
Are there any television programmes and personalities you particularly like
or dislike? *(Give details.)*

_____

_____

_____

Radio
Are there any programmes and personalities you particularly like or dislike?
(Give details.)

_____

_____

_____

Personal Communication History Form ...continued

Music

Are you interested in any particular kinds of music? *(Give details.)*

_____

_____

Did/do you sing, play an instrument, etc? *(Give details.)*

_____

_____

_____

Reading

Did you read a newspaper regularly before your illness? ☐ Yes ☐ No
(If so, which one?)

_____

_____

Do/did you read any magazines regularly? ☐ Yes ☐ No
(If so, which ones?)

_____

_____

_____

Do you have any favourite books or authors?

_____

_____

_____

Sociability

Please rate the following activities (from 1 to 4) in order of the client's preference.

Spending time alone	☐	Meeting new people	☐
Spending time with relatives	☐	Spending time with friends	☐

Interests

Can you think of anything else we should know about you that might stimulate your interest, bring back memories, and generally help to encourage communication?

_____

_____

_____

Personal Communication History Form ...continued

4 Effects of the medical condition

What sort of a person were you before the illness *(eg, quiet, talkative, anxious, humorous, lively, short-tempered, thoughtful …)*? *(Please give as much information as possible as this will affect the direction of therapy.)*

_____

_____

_____

Do you feel your behaviour has changed since the illness?
(Please give details.)

_____

_____

_____

Do you ever feel 'why me?' in relation to your present condition?

_____

_____

_____

If you are physically disabled in any way, as a result of the illness, what do you feel, if anything, about this?

_____

_____

_____

Is there any specific activity that you are no longer able to carry out, which causes you particular anxiety/distress?

_____

_____

_____

Can you think of anything else we should know that might be of interest, help bring back memories, or help encourage your communication?

_____

_____

_____

Thank you for the time it has taken you to complete this questionnaire.

Why Relax?

Name _____ Date _____

Life today can be very fast-moving, with many demands upon our time. It is easy to hurry from task to task without realising the effect of stress and strain.

If you are the type of person who tries to do everything in the shortest time, or becomes irritated when things do not happen when you want, because you are reliant on others, you are likely to make yourself tense and over tired.

Some people find that they become irritable when they are doing nothing, or if they are unable to do things for themselves. You may notice that your neck and shoulders feel stiff and painful. This tension can affect the voice. Tension is one way your body can tell you to slow down and relax.

Relaxation should always be part of your way of life, whether you are sitting down doing nothing, or carrying out your normal day-to-day activities. Relaxation is important because, if you are relaxed, your voice and speech will be easier.

Trying to relax

Initially, you need to find situations, or to think about situations that you personally find relaxing. Different scenarios work for different people, so you need to think about what suits you.

Situations
Examples include:
◆ Sitting in a darkened, quiet room
◆ Listening to soft, relaxing music
◆ Being in the room in which you feel most comfortable.

Why Relax? ...*continued*

Thoughts

Examples include:

◆ A sandy beach with the sea lapping on the shore

◆ Sitting in a field overlooking a pretty village

◆ Sitting by a river

◆ A winter scene in front of an open log fire.

What can stop you relaxing?

It is important to be aware of those situations that make you tense – for example, shopping, people being late, being unable to do certain activities others are participating in. Becoming aware of when you are 'tense', and what that feels like, will help you to know how to feel relaxed.

How to relax

Breathing tends to become shallow when we are anxious, nervous, tense or excited, as our heart rate increases.

Relaxation and a strong resonant voice require controlled, regular breathing with an adequate air supply. This results in a slowing down of the heart rate. The maximum potential for expansion of the lungs is at the base of the lungs, where rib movement is less restricted. Posture needs to be as erect as you are personally able to achieve, to allow good expansion. This also helps to overcome any tendency to raise the shoulders in an attempt to increase lung capacity.

If you are able, begin by putting your hand(s) on your lower rib-cage and watch yourself in a mirror.

◆ Breathe in slowly and feel your chest swell up with air.

◆ Hold for a second and then squeeze it out. Your stomach muscles should be relaxed while your rib-cage is 'swelling up', and tight when they push the air out.

◆ Do this five times.

Doing this exercise will help you become aware of the rhythm of your breathing pattern.

Sourcebook for Assessing & Maintaining Communication
© F Sugden-Best 2002

Are You a Relaxed Person?

Name _____ Date _____

The following set of questions is designed to evaluate your reactions to potential situations that may be stressful. Being stressed can have an effect on our communication skills. Tick all those that apply.

1 I often wake up tired after a good night's sleep. ☐

2 I easily become impatient waiting for things to be done. ☐

3 I can easily lose my temper when others do not understand me. ☐

4 I tend to interrupt others, rather than waiting for them to finish what they are saying. ☐

5 I often jump at sudden noises. ☐

6 People get on my nerves if they are around me all the time. ☐

7 I dislike crowded rooms and places. ☐

8 I think at length about my illness. ☐

Total /8

Head, Neck and Shoulders Relaxation

Handout
34
© F Sugden-Best 2002

Name _____ Date _____

These are general exercises to help relax the head, neck and shoulders. Sit in a comfortable position, with your feet on the ground or foot plates of your wheelchair, if applicable. Do each exercise three to five times, relaxing between each movement. Correct your position between movements, if required. Do the exercises slowly, three times a day, and when you are feeling at all tense.

1 Starting with your head in the mid-position, resting towards your chest, slowly move your head to the left, to the mid-point, to the right, to the mid-point.

2 Move your chin slowly down towards your chest, then back to the normal position.

3 Move your head slowly to look over your right shoulder. Repeat to the left. Turn only as far as is comfortable each time, to feel the pull of your muscles.

4 Imagine the tip of your nose is a pencil. Slowly draw small circles in the air in front of you, moving towards the left, and then to the right.

5 Rotate your shoulders forwards, slowly making a full circle. Repeat, moving your shoulders backwards. You can also do this exercise one shoulder at a time.

6 Lift your shoulders up once, and from this point lift your shoulders slightly higher. Release your shoulders.

7 Gradually try to bring your shoulders together in front of you; then move them back to their normal position.

8 Gradually try to push your shoulders backwards; then back to their normal position.

Why is Posture Important for Speech and Voice Production?

Name _____ Date _____

The clarity of your speech and quality of your voice can be affected by your ability to use adequate breath support. Poor posture can result from muscular weakness, and it can be more difficult to achieve this support when in a sitting position.

Common problems can be:

◆ **Tension**

◆ **Slumping** – where the rib-cage sinks in towards the pelvis, and the spine is rounded. This can affect the efficiency of breathing.

◆ **Rounded shoulders**

◆ **Pushing the torso upwards and forwards** – like a sergeant major. This encourages shallow breathing.

◆ **Shoulders raised** – towards the ears and pushed inwards to the neck. This produces tension in the throat.

◆ **Head pulled back** – again causing excessive neck tension.

Let's Breathe

Name _____ Date _____

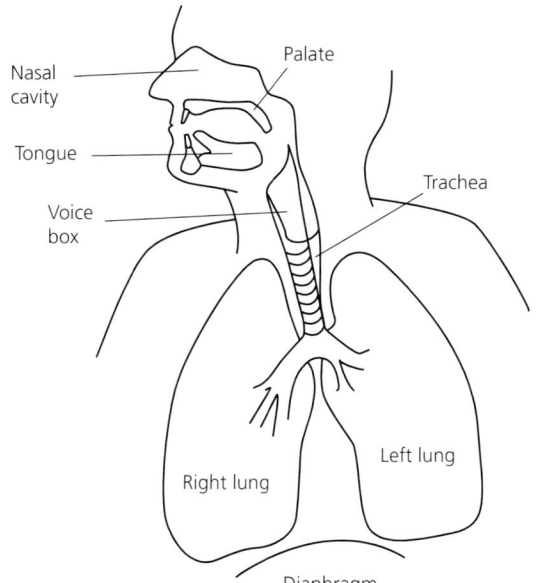

A good supply of air and effective breath control are important for the clear articulation of speech sounds, and for control of the loudness of the voice. They are also important for emphasis and the rhythm of speech.

Your lungs are like a pair of bellows that pump air out through your voice box – that is, larynx – making your vocal cords vibrate to produce voice. Good breathing is supported by the abdominal muscles and by the diaphragm. When breathing correctly, the shoulders should not be tense or raised, and the upper chest should not move.

To begin, sit in a quiet room, preferably in front of a mirror, and concentrate on what happens to your body as you gently breathe in and out. Watch your rib-cage and stomach moving in and out. Breathe in through your nose, so that the air is partially warmed and particles such as dirt are trapped on the hair follicles, and breathe out through your mouth. It is important to be aware of your normal breathing pattern at rest before altering it in any way.

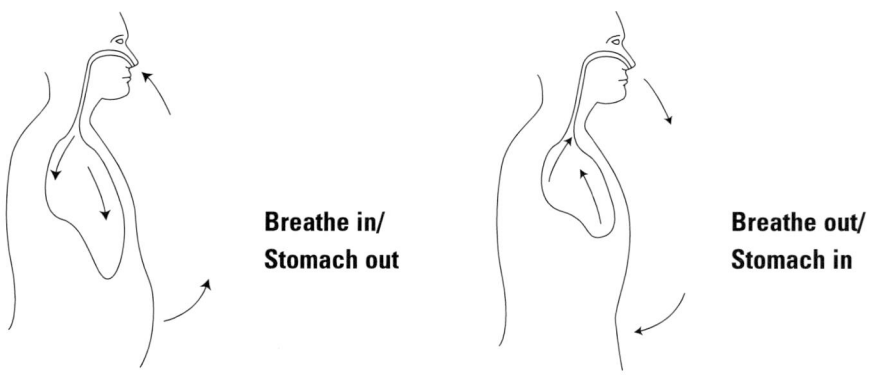

**Breathe in/
Stomach out**

**Breathe out/
Stomach in**

The following exercises are designed to aid diaphragmatic breathing. Do each one three times, taking a rest between movements. If you become out of breath, stop. Do the exercises in stages.

Before starting any of the following exercises, make sure you are sitting in a comfortable chair that supports you well, in a quiet room. Relax your trunk, your shoulders, your neck, and your head.

Remember the aims of the exercises are:
◆ To establish the correct type of breathing pattern
◆ To increase the capacity of the lungs
◆ To control inhalation and exhalation of air

Breathing Exercises

Name _____ Date _____

1 Take in a deep breath. Release the air comfortably until you begin to run out. Practise releasing the air and counting the length of time you are breathing out. If possible keep a record of this information by using the second-hand on your watch.

2 Breathe in to a silent count of two. Hold your breath for two. Breathe out to a silent count of two. If this felt comfortable, count to three.

3 Breathe in and breathe out saying a series of 'ha's, using the following patterns. Top up with breath as required.

    – means a short 'ha'
    —— means a long 'ha'

    —— –   —— –   —— –

    – ——   – ——   – ——

    – – ——   – – ——   – – ——

4 When breathing out, pretend you are blowing out a candle, expelling all the air from your lungs. Repeat.

5 Take a deep breath. Release the air on two equal puffs. Gradually build up to release the air on three, four and then five equal puffs, if able.

6 Take a breath in and count out loud slowly up to three. Gradually increase up to ten, if possible, on one breath.

7 Take a deep breath in. Hold and let the breath out on a long 'sss' sound. Count to yourself how long the sound continues.

8 Take a deep breath in and practise getting gradually louder – that is, crescendo – on 'ss'.

9 Take a deep breath in and practise getting gradually softer – that is, diminuendo – on 'ss'.

10 Take a deep breath in and practise flowing from louder to softer – that is, gliding on 'ss'.

11 Take a deep breath in. Release the air using different rhythmical patterns.

—— means long blow out
– means short blow out

—— —— — –   —— —— — –   —— —— — –

– – ——   – – ——   – – ——

—— —— – – —— —— – – —— —— – –

12 Breathe in, counting silently up to three, then breathe out on:

pa pa pa pa	ba ba ba ba	ta ta ta ta
da da da da	ga ga ga ga	sa sa sa sa
za za za za	ma ma ma ma	na na na na
wa wa wa wa	sha sha sha sha	ja ja ja ja

Voice Exercises 1

Name _____ Date _____

Following on from the breathing exercises:

1 Sing different vowels on one unbroken, evenly sustained breath.

'ah' .... 'oo' .... 'ee' ....

Then sing continuously, moving from one vowel to another.

'ah' → 'oo' → 'ee' → 'oh'

2 Sing vowels, with a pause between each one.

'ah' ... stop → 'oo' ... stop → 'ee' ...

Produce on one sustained breath.

3 Make a gentle sound before the vowel glide into voicing.

fffff → ahhhhhhhhh
sss → eeeeeeeeee
sh → oooooooooo

4 Practise humming – that is, 'mmm' – feeling the vibration on your lips.

5 Practise humming to vowels, moving up and down the scale.

'mmm' → 'ah' 'mmm' → 'ah' 'mmm' → 'ah'
 ♫ high note ♫ medium note ♫ low note

6 Practise humming to vowels in rapid succession. This helps to develop use of nasal resonance.

'mmm' → 'ah' → 'mmm' → 'ah' → 'mmm'
'mmm' → 'oo' → 'mmm' → 'oo' → 'mmm'

7 Move between voiceless – that is, not using the vocal cords – and voiced sounds – that is, using the vocal cords in repetitive strings.

fvfvfvfvfvfvfvfvfvf

szszszszszszszs

Voice Exercises 2

Name _____ Date _____

The aims of these voice exercises are to:
- ◆ Establish coordination of breathing out and producing voice
- ◆ Achieve good vocal quality
- ◆ Control vocal volume
- ◆ Help vary pitch and inflection
- ◆ Achieve good resonance.

1 Sigh out on a soft, breathy 'h' sound, then follow with a vowel sound, for example:

h → ah   h → ee

h → oh   h → aw

2 Gradually reduce the length of the breathy 'h' and increase the length of the vowel sound, for example:

h…ah………   h…ee………

3 Say other sounds before the vowel sounds, for example:

p → ah   sh → ah
f → oo   sh → ay

4 Gradually increase the length of the vowel sounds compared to the other sound, for example:

p.. ee………   f.. ah………..

5 Glide from one vowel to another, for example:

ah → oo → ee
oo → ah → aw

6 (a) Hum, holding on to the sound 'mmm' as long as possible.

(b) Say 'm' followed by a vowel. For example:

m → ah   m → oh

(c) Repeat (b) in a sequence. For example:

mah → mee → mah
may → maw → moo

7 Sing up and down the scale to 'lah' or 'mmm'. For example:

♫ 'lah' low   ♫ 'lah' middle ♫ 'lah' high
♫ 'lah' high ♫ 'lah' middle ♫ 'lah' low

8 Say the vowel sound 'ah' or 'oh' with a changing intonation pattern – that is, with a change in pitch. For example:

'ah'	↗	Rising inflection
'ah'	↘	Falling inflection
'ah'	∧	Rise/fall
'ah'	∨	Fall/rise

Soft, Easy Voice

Name _____ Date _____

These exercises give you guidelines on how best to produce your voice without excessive tension and effort.

Things to remember:

1 Make sure you're relaxed. If possible, go through your relaxation exercises before working on this set of exercises.

2 Throughout the exercises, make sure you have enough breath to support the production of your voice.

3 Practise the exercises in a quiet room where you are unlikely to be disturbed.

4 Monitor yourself when you produce voice:
   ◆ Do you force your voice out?
   ◆ Do you tense up your shoulders/neck/facial muscles?
   ◆ Does your voice sound harsh and strained?
   ◆ Does your breath run out while you're producing voice?
   ◆ Does your volume vary?
   ◆ Does your voice sound faltering and weak?

During the exercises, aim for a gentle, smooth voice, produced without tension in your shoulders, neck, face or chest. Make sure you always have enough air to support your voice. If you run out of breath during the exercises, stop and start again.

Soft, Easy Voice Exercises

Name _____ Date _____

1 Begin by sighing out gently, and then glide smoothly into the following vowels:

sigh ⟶ ah
sigh ⟶ oo
sigh ⟶ ee
sigh ⟶ oh

Remember to stop if you hear your voice faltering, or if it sounds hoarse and strained.

2 Repeat Exercise 1 above, producing a hum:

hmmm ⟶ ah
hmmm ⟶ oo
hmmm ⟶ ee
hmmm ⟶ oh

During this exercise, hum very gently. Try to feel the vibrations in your lips, as you open and close your mouth, while humming continuously.

3 Remembering the sensation you experienced in Exercise 2, now practise with short words.
For example:

him	ma	hoe	me
her	more	how	moo
he	mare	high	my

4 During the following phrases, try to run the words together to keep your voice sounding smooth. Remember to look out for signs that your breath is running out:

How are you?	'hahwahyoo'
Who are you?	'hooahyoo'
Where are you?	'hwereahyoo'

Who is he?	How is it?
Where is home?	How high is it?
Home sweet home.	Herbert is home.
Where is Mark?	When was he here?

Breath Control Exercises

Name _____ Date _____

The aim of these exercises is to extend breath control in order to say sentences of increasing length.

Remember to take a good breath of air before each sentence. Gradually release your breath. Do not release all the air at the beginning, otherwise you will not have enough air to complete each sentence.

1   Three.
Thirty-three.
Thirty-three times.
Thirty-three times ten.
Thirty-three times ten is three hundred and thirty.

2   She jumped.
She jumped high.
She jumped high and long.
She jumped high, long and completely.
She jumped high, long, completely and fully.

3 John went away.
John went away to France.
John went away to France yesterday.
John went away to France yesterday for
    a week.
John went away to France yesterday for
    a week to stay with friends.

4 I want a dog.
I want a brown dog.
I want a brown, long-haired dog.
I want a brown, long-haired dog with
    big feet.
I want a brown, long-haired dog with
    big feet and floppy ears.

Pitch Exercises

Name _____ Date _____

1 Humming any tune, listen to the various notes you can produce.

2 Continue humming the tune, but stop at various points and count from 1 to 5 on the same note.

3 Sing a tune on the following vowel sounds:

oo   ah   aw   ah   ee

4 Using the same vowels, speak one on a high pitch, one on a middle pitch and one on a low pitch. Say them with a softly produced 'h' in front.

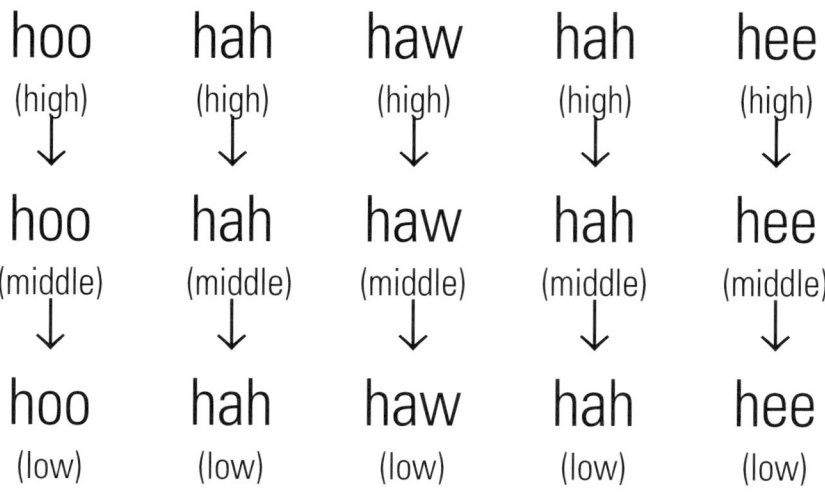

hoo	hah	haw	hah	hee
(high)	(high)	(high)	(high)	(high)
↓	↓	↓	↓	↓
hoo	hah	haw	hah	hee
(middle)	(middle)	(middle)	(middle)	(middle)
↓	↓	↓	↓	↓
hoo	hah	haw	hah	hee
(low)	(low)	(low)	(low)	(low)

5 Repeat Exercise 4, but begin on the low note and travel up to the high note:

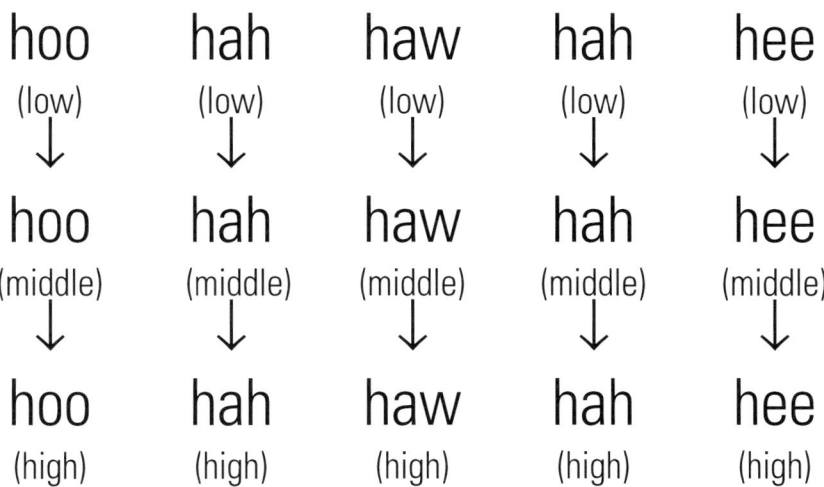

hoo	hah	haw	hah	hee
(low)	(low)	(low)	(low)	(low)
↓	↓	↓	↓	↓
hoo	hah	haw	hah	hee
(middle)	(middle)	(middle)	(middle)	(middle)
↓	↓	↓	↓	↓
hoo	hah	haw	hah	hee
(high)	(high)	(high)	(high)	(high)

6 Speak the following, taking a new, higher pitch note for each word:

                                                higher
                                          and
                                    higher
                              climb
                        voice
                  my
            make
      can
I

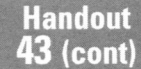

7   Speak the following, taking a new, lower pitch note for each word:

I
    can
        make
            my
                voice
                    go
                        lower
                            and
                                lower

Pitch Diagrams

Name _____ Date _____

1 Crescendo

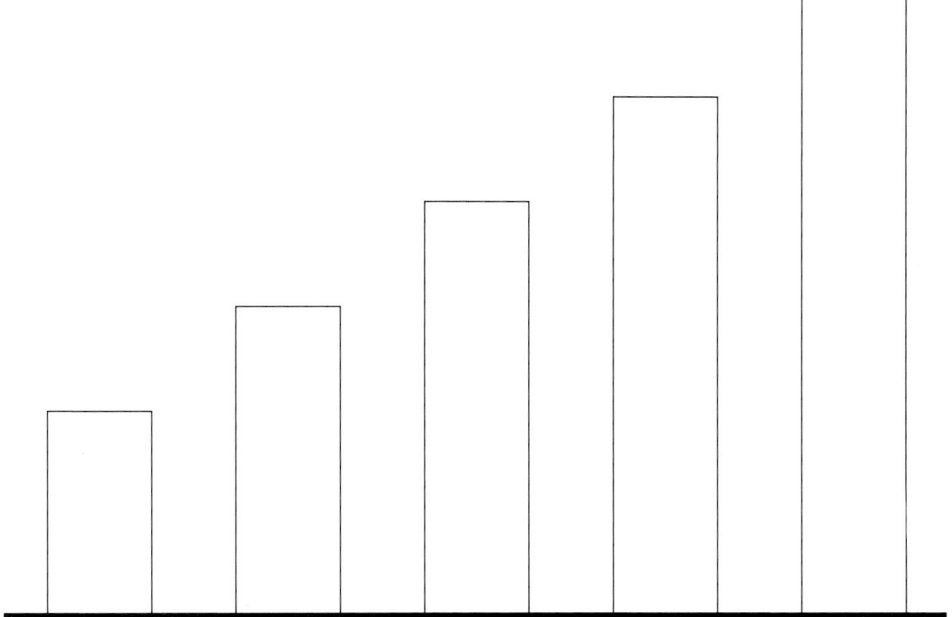

2 Diminuendo

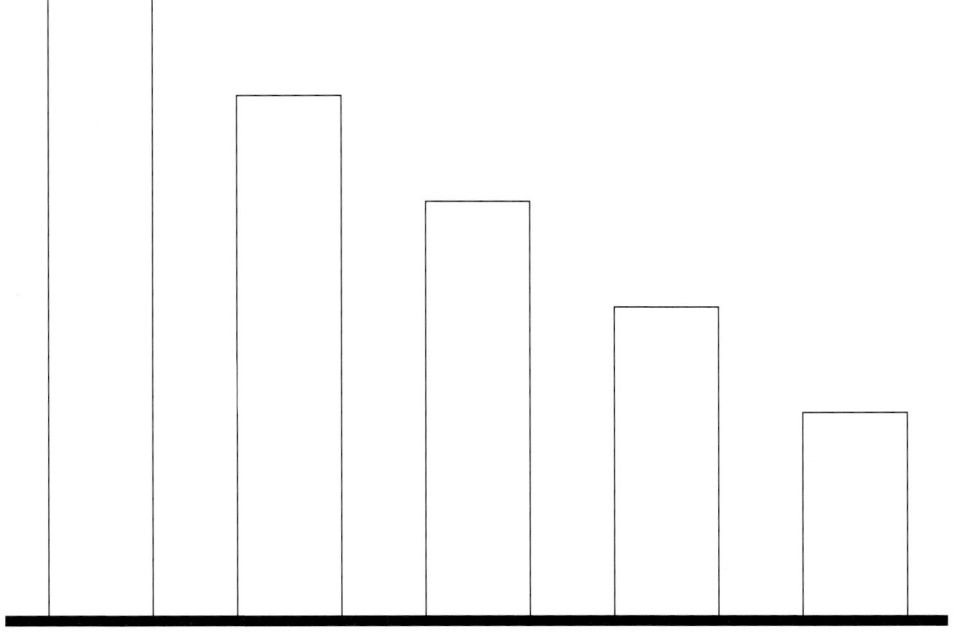

Pitch Diagrams

Name _____ Date _____

3 Crescendo/diminuendo

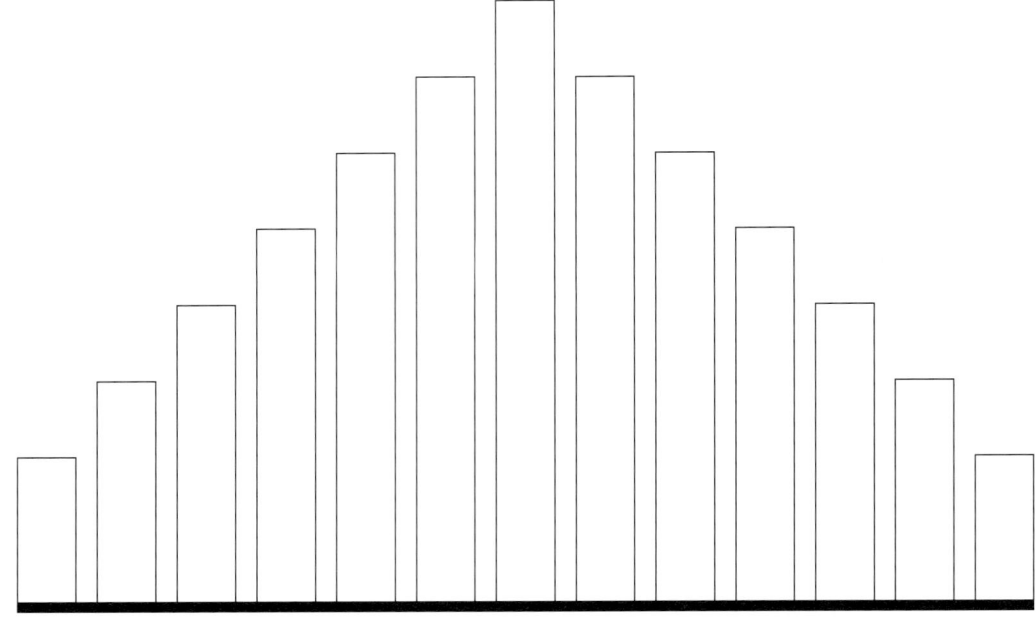

4 Diminuendo/crescendo

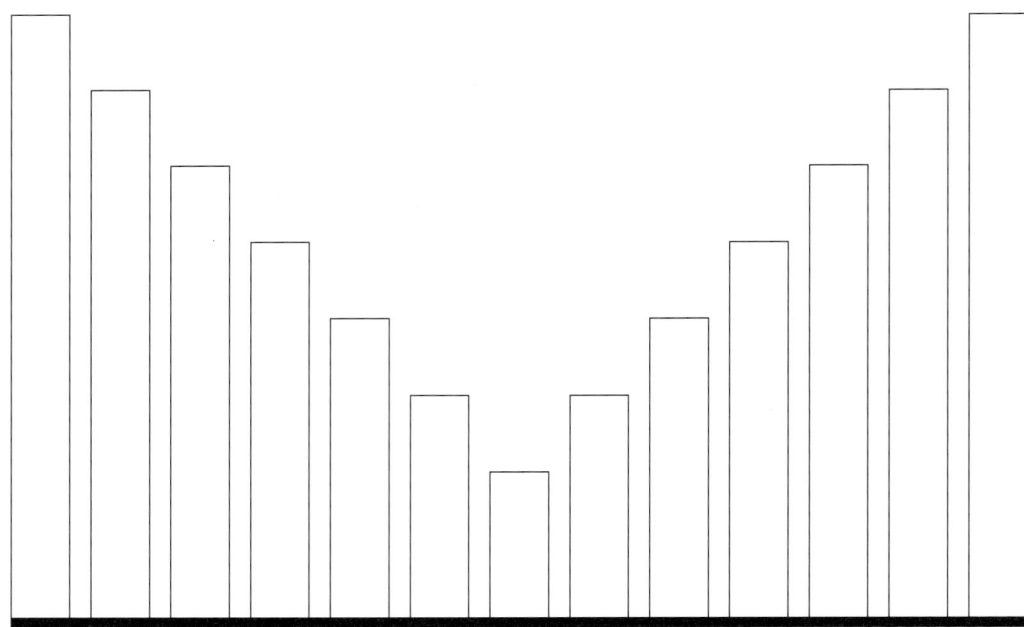

Pitch Diagrams

Name _____ Date _____

5   Pitch jumps

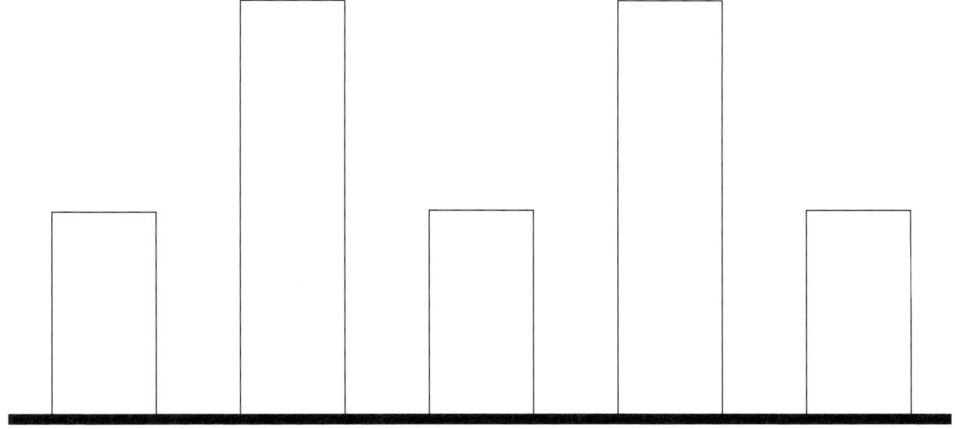

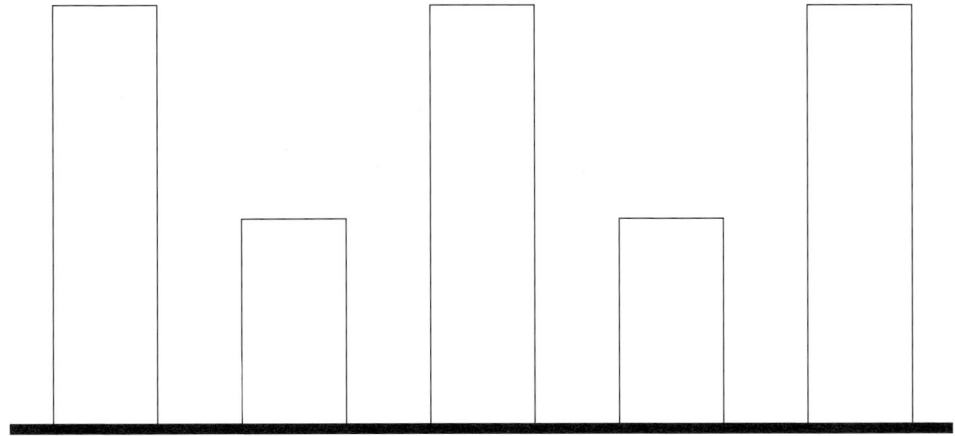

Intonation Exercises

Name _____ Date _____

1 Practise intonation patterns on 'ah'.

'ah' ↗ move from low to high ▬ ■

'ah' ↘ move from high to low ■ ▬

'ah' ⋀ move from low to high
to low ▬ ■ ▬

'ah' ⋁ move from high to low
to high ■ ▬ ■

2 Repeat, using the word 'oh'.

3 Repeat, using the word 'why'.

4 Repeat, using the word 'no'.

5 Try to convey different emotions using 'oh' and 'why.' For example:

Excited   Bored   Happy
Sad   Angry   Frustrated
Sarcastic

6 Practise the following sentences, all with a rising intonation pattern on the last word, that is ↗ ▬ ■

Do you want chips? Are you happy?
Is this your dog? Do you swim?

7 Practise the following sentences, all with a falling intonation pattern on the last word, that is ↘ ■ ▬

You may be right. Don't say any more.
Please sit down. I'm very unhappy.

8 Try to use intonation in the following sentences.

How are you? I am fed up.
I like this. You let me down.
What do you mean? Is it time?
Let's go home.

9 Think about how you may be able to change the meaning or mood conveyed in the following sentences by changing the intonation pattern.

Are you ready?
What do you mean?
I'm really enjoying myself.
Whatever you want.

Why do Resonance Exercises?

Name _____ Date _____

Your voice is produced by breath passing up through your vocal cords in your voice box (larynx), causing them to vibrate. The sound waves created are then modified as they pass up through your throat, mouth and nose.

Resonance refers to the way in which these cavities vibrate (resonate), just as a musical instrument does, to shape and project each individual sound.

These exercises are designed to alter the focus of your voice, so that you will be able to project your voice more effectively.

The sounds 'm' and 'n' are nasal sounds. This is because the air comes down your nose as well as out of your mouth. This means you should be able to feel your nasal area vibrating if you prolong either of the sounds.

Resonance Exercises 1

Name _____ Date _____

Repeat each exercise five times, relaxing between each movement.

1 Breathe in, hold, and breathe out to an easy hum – that is, 'mmm'.

You should be able to feel a gentle vibration of your nose and your mouth. Try to send the sound forward, so your lips tingle, and maintain an easy relaxed throat.

Use a pitch that is easy to maintain. Be aware of sustaining a constant sound quality. The quality will change noticeably when you begin to run out of air.

2 Take a deep breath. Produce a 'hmm' in two equal portions – that is, with a breath between each 'hmm'. If able:

◆ Produce a 'hmm' in three equal portions.
◆ Produce a 'hmm' in four equal portions.
◆ Produce a 'hmm' in five equal portions.

3 Produce a number of little 'hmm', 'hmm', 'hmm's.

4 Practise humming, starting off quietly and then seeing if you can gradually become louder – that is, crescendo:

'mmm' 'mmm' 'mmm' 'mmm' 'mmm'.

5 Practise humming, starting off loudly and then seeing if you can gradually become softer – that is, diminuendo:

'mmm' 'mmm' 'mmm' 'mmm' 'mmm'.

6 Take a deep breath. Produce a gentle 'mmm' while you count to five to yourself, then six, then seven.

7 Sustain the humming sound. See if you can glide up and down the scale, keeping the quality of the sound as even as possible. It does not matter if the loudness or volume changes, focus on the quality of the sound you produce.

8 Produce your 'mmm's in rhythmical patterns, for example:

'mmm' = long   'mm' = short

'mmm' 'mm'   'mmm' 'mm'   'mmm' 'mm'
'mm' 'mmm'   'mm' 'mmm'   'mm' 'mmm'
'mm' 'mm' 'mmm'   'mm' 'mm' 'mmm'   'mm' 'mm' 'mmm'

9 Hum, followed by a vowel sound, for example:

'mmm' 'ah'
'mmm' 'oo'

10 As you say 'm' plus the vowel, try to move up the scale and then down the scale as you produce each sound combination, for example:

'moo' – high note ♫ medium note ♫ low note ♫
              low note ♫ medium note ♫ high note ♫

Repeat for 'me', 'may', 'more', etc.

Resonance Exercises 2

Name _____ Date _____

1 Say two short words one after the other
 – that is, 'm' + a vowel. For example:

Moo + Me	Me + Moo
May + Moo	Mum + May
May + My	Mine + Me
Mum + May	Might + More

2 Try several short words one after the
 other. For example:

 Moo + Me + My + More
 May + More + Might + Mum
 More + May + Mint + Man

3 Repeat the above exercises using 'n'
 instead of 'm'. For example:

 No + Knee + Nice + New

4 Try some short words and phrases:

meat – Have some meat.
neat – He is neat.

man – Be the man.
nan – How is your nan?

moon – The moon is out.
noon – It is now noon.

mine – It is mine.
nine – Nine pills.

5 Hum, followed by a day of the week.
For example:

'mmm' → Monday
'mmm' → Tuesday

6 Hum, followed by a month of the year.
For example:

'mmm' → January
'mmm' → April

7 Say the days of the week without a hum.

8 Say the months of the year without a hum.

9 Count in groups of numbers, topping up with air in between each group. For example:

1, 2, 3 pause, 4, 5, 6 pause, 7, 8, 9

Gradually increase the groups of numbers. For example :

2, 3, 4, 5 pause.

Chapter 3

Articulation Sheets

This chapter contains stimulation word lists for the dysarthric speaker. These are designed to be photocopied for direct use. The size and type of font have been chosen with the needs of those with visual impairment in mind.

These sheets can be particularly useful for clients with Motor Neurone disease and Multiple System Atrophy, for example, who fatigue quickly, where the focus of articulatory work needs to be on functional usage. Concentrating on non-speech-related activities can be unnecessarily tiring and counter-productive. Specific words can be chosen from the lists in order to concentrate on either problem sounds or regularly used/problem words.

◆ A selection of multisyllabic words is provided for each individual sound. Consonant clusters have also been included on separate pages, with stimulation words for initial, medial and final positions, as appropriate. Certain sounds or consonant clusters can be selected for specific practice.

◆ There are lists of tongue-twister sentences for the higher-level dysarthric speaker, with consonant clusters often being included in the list for a particular sound. For example, 'b', 'bl' and 'br' sheets are included for words of two to six syllables and sentences of three to seven syllables. A final list of multisyllabic sentences, each of which contains a number of multisyllabic words, is also provided.

Some clients are happy to incorporate list-reading into their standard exercise programmes. The clinician can use tape recording and encourage the development of self-monitoring skills. If working with a carer or volunteer, sentences can be made up for some of the words, with the client having to articulate the missing word clearly, thus enabling the same stimulation words to be used. For example:

Therapist: 'When the bin is full you take out the _____.'
Patient: 'Rubbish.'

The client should be made aware of the specific sound currently being worked on, so that it may be given particular attention.

B – Multisyllabic Words

baboonish	backbiter
burdening	backbencher
bamboozle	basketball
barbiturate	buckboard
bilberry	bobbysock
bendable	bombastic
booby-trap	bumble-bee
bombard	believable

blow	blackberry
blue	blissfully
black	blitheness
blade	blackmarket
blob	blunderbuss
bloom	blue pencil
blobby	blood-transfusion
bluster	blamelessly

Initial	*Medial*	*Final*
brown	library	n/a
brush	abroad	
brass	abridge	
brook	algebra	
bread	calibre	
broken	umbrella	
brother	celebrate	
bristle	labrador	

BR – Multisyllabic Words

celebration	brainstorm
brazeness	brandy-snap
umbrageous	bricklayer
librarianship	brotherliness
brilliantly	brother-in-law
brushwood	vibratory
bristliness	broadminded
algebraist	abridgment

The buds on the bare boughs are about to burst into blossom.

Robin redbreast bobbed about begging for crumbs.

Bluebeard, the brute, murdered a bevy of beautiful blondes.

There was a buzzing of buzy bees in the bushes and blossom.

A bold bandit broke into the bank and robbed it of its best bonds.

In his big, black car was a box full of bargain books.

I believe Beryl has bought a big box of brandy balls.

Brian was broadminded and brought a brooch for Brenda.

Blue and black blowflies are blind.

Beware of Bob who blows up umbrellas when bathing.

P – Multisyllabic Words

palpable	palpitate
papering	palmiped
panoply	puppetry
participate	participle
perpetrate	perception
pomposity	popularity
pot-pourri	perpetual

Initial	Medial	Final
plain	reply	apple
place	replace	ample
play	imply	
plot	comply	
plant	display	
plateau	complain	
plastic	complete	
plaster	deplete	

Handout
56
© F Sugden-Best 2002

implication	plasterboard
plagiarism	planetarium
plain-speaking	plasticity
complication	plantation
plesiosaurus	plenipotentiary
complementary	plutonium
plutocratic	pleasurable

Initial	Medial	Final
prop	express	n/a
prune	impress	
pray	appraise	
prose	reprint	
press	improve	
princess	repress	
prison	approve	
practise	compress	

PR – Multisyllabic Words

improvisation	practicability
pragmatism	reproduction
precipitate	predicament
predecessor	comprehensively
appreciative	preservation
preselective	profundity
preponderance	apprehensibility

Poor Peter was pummelled and punched till purple.

Some people prefer prunes to plums and apples.

Pingpong is a popular sport played in many places.

Portugal, Peru and Persia are far apart.

He painted a picture of penguins playing on a purple pond.

The pretty pet performs plenty of pleasant tricks.

Plastic and plasterboard are plainly of poor quality.

Prue praised Peter for his practicability and prudence.

Some people prefer applying pleasurable pressure to pain.

When shopping she purchased apples, parsnips and pizzas.

M – Multisyllabic Words

mammal

matrimony

marshmallow

maladministration

marjoram

mechanism

monochrome

macramé

magnesium

mannerism

mammoth

marmoset

momentary

myxomatosis

M – Tongue-Twisters

The murmur of bees in elms brought back memories of summers.

There are many monks in the monasteries in Rome.

Some men may make mistakes in mathematics.

He made an immense amount of money making ammunitions.

Make those men move smartly, Major!

The room filled with the musty smell of mouldering melons.

Mary and Myrtle were merry maids.

Who smashed every mug in the mansion?

Simon makes a practice of smothering meat in mustard.

Maureen was impressed by Mum's method of mashing.

T – Multisyllabic Words

tabulate	tactical
tail-light	talkative
terrestrial	tessellated
tantamount	teleprinter
typewriter	temperate
tetanus	titmouse
totalitarian	turntable

Initial	Medial	Final
try	entrap	n/a
true	retrace	
trip	retrain	
trot	entrance	
tray	nitric	
trolley	retry	
trailer	ashtray	
traffic	retread	

TR – Multisyllabic Words

nitroglycerine	traditional
trajectory	tranquillity
transcendence	retractable
transformation	intransitive
transitional	treasonable
transubstantiation	contradictory
contravention	transparency

twin	twaddler
tweet	tweaking
twirl	twentieth
twist	twittering
twitch	tweezers
twang	twenty

T – Tongue-Twisters

The ten, tiny tots were taught by a tutor from Eton.

The train trip took a tiresome twenty-two hours.

Tim tore his trousers and lost two buttons.

Tell Thomas to take a turn at table tennis.

Too many teenagers waste time watching television.

The still torpid tortoise put out a tentative foot.

Terry trapped Tim, his twin, in terrible traffic.

The trout was toasted by Tina for Tom's tea.

The tractor turned to the right and trampled twenty tulips.

To tell the truth is tempting in times of trouble.

dachshund	dandelion
deaden	decadence
deciduous	dedicate
dependable	desperado
duodenum	didactic
diffidently	dedicated
dilapidated	diminuendo

DR

Initial	Medial	Final
dry	redress	n/a
drop	address	
drain	eardrum	
dress	doldrums	
droop	teardrop	
drum	mandrill	
dresser	mandrel	
dreamy	adrift	

dragon-fly	dramatisation
dramaturgy	draughtsmanship
drawbridge	dressmaker
drowsiness	dry-saltery
drunkenness	dressing-room
dropsical	dromedary

D – Tongue-Twisters

A deep ditch divides the meadow from the dwelling.

Don't dare meddle with documents in the drawer.

Dennie's daughter Diana doesn't dislike darning.

I dared the dastard to a dreadful duel.

It's dangerous to deal with a daring bandit.

Don't do as I do, or you'll do what it isn't done to do!

He didn't dare saddle the dangerous donkey.

Douglas and Derek were due at Diana's for dinner on Monday.

The dragon-fly delighted the dachshund by dwelling in his eardrum.

The guard was hiding under the window on Monday.

L – Multisyllabic Words

lacteal	landlady
lanolin	laconically
laughable	legality
legislature	liberally
lilliputian	listlessly
livelihood	luckless
luxuriantly	loneliness

L – Tongue-Twisters

Let Lucy light a candle to look for the blue ball.

A little pill will cure a great ill.

Poor little Billie is so silly, she's almost a liability.

He lost his life in the struggle for liberty.

The foolish fellow left his wallet lying on the table.

Molehills in the fields show moles making tunnels in the soil.

He lay on the luxurious pillow listening to the landlady laughing loudly.

The silly lad longed to lend Linda his yellow umbrella.

Will it take long for the hole to fill with coloured leaves?

N – Multisyllabic Words

banana	napkin
nationally	nervousness
nicotine	nightingale
nonagenarian	nondescript
nonsense	nominee
notwithstanding	pneumonia
notification	nonsensical

N – Tongue-Twisters

© F Sugden-Best 2002

Doesn't anyone know where the new knives are?

There were nine nice nasturtiums in a line.

That fine bunch of bananas will make a nice snack for noon.

The green and lemon napkins are never neat.

There are no poisonous snakes anywhere near here.

To never take snuff means you'll sneeze noisily.

The naughty panda ran to join the winner.

Nancy is a nurse but nobody can handle her darning.

The widow was too nervous to have dinner with William.

Nothing is nicer than runny honey on bananas.

R – Multisyllabic Words

rapturous	rarefaction
rarity	raspberry
reboring	recuperate
regenerate	reserve
rarify	respirator
restaurant	reverted
resurrection	reverberate

R – Tongue-Twisters

Those are really pretty red roses.

The Reverend Roper arrived from Rome three days ago.

Harris rarely reads literary reviews.

The real reason is really rather curious.

The merry drummer drank more ale than was right.

She wore a red dress of a rough, rusty-red material.

In Harrods, Ruth bought marrows, carrots, cherries and oranges.

Rachel read the story regarding the fairy and the earring.

Tomorrow, I will borrow a really rustic barrow from Ralph.

wallaby	wanderer
wardrobe	wastefully
watchmaker	watermark
weariness	welcoming
wellington	westward
welterweight	willingness
windward	workmanship
worshipper	

W – Tongue-Twisters

Wee Willie wept wildly as his wicked uncle whipped him.

Which word would one want, if one wanted a word?

A weird white wolf wandered wearily into the wood.

'What will you wear, a white waistcoat or a woollen sweater?'

What, why, when and where are words we use when we want to ask questions.

The quality of woollen wares is well worth looking into.

We always wander to the watchmakers when away in Wales.

The workmanship of the wardrobe was well below standard.

The wolf and the wasp were washing in the window of the woman's wagon.

F – Multisyllabic Words

fabricate	facsimile
fitfully	faithfully
falsetto	fandango
farthingale	favourable
fearlessly	fulfilment
figurative	footfault
fermentation	forefinger

fly	flamingo
flow	flabbergasted
fling	flamboyant
flit	flannelette
float	fluidity
flash	fledgling
fluffy	fleetingly
flower	fluorescence

free	frostbite
fry	friability
fresh	friendliness
fret	frightfulness
frog	freemasonry
friend	frankfurter
frolic	frankincense
frosty	frustration

F – Tongue-Twisters

Five fine fellows met at four on the first of February.

'Philip,' said Ferdinand, 'I fear we must fight.'

Philip fought fairly for fifty-five minutes.

The furry fox quaffed a tankard of frothy beer.

Francis felt fat and foolish after toffees and coffee.

After the friends finished fretting, they left to fish.

Half a loaf and four figs were finished by Fred on Friday.

It was foul and frosty in Florida at five fifty.

Phil was awful to Francis following the festival at the farm.

vaccinate	vagabond
vandalism	vaporisation
vegetarianism	ventilate
vermicelli	versatility
vestibule	veterinary
victimise	virtuoso
vol-au-vent	vulnerable

V – Tongue-Twisters

Vice shall not vanquish virtue.

The villainous Vivian visited the village.

The various efforts to evade the knight were in vain.

Sir Oliver vaulted on to his horse and veered down the valley.

The valiant Vernon vowed to discover the villain's cave.

A diver was saved by Vera who isn't even clever.

Violets were waving on the veranda of Veronica's house.

Every van is ventilated via a very lovely ventilator.

Eleven violins and violas were vandalised by a very violent driver.

TH – Multisyllabic Words

thankful	thallium
theatrical	thaumaturge
theology	theodolite
theoretical	therapeutic
thermostat	thermometer
thermodynamics	thixotropic
thrombosis	threshold

three

thrall

threw

thresh

throw

thrift

throaty

threadbare

threnodial

thrombosis

threshold

TH – Tongue-Twisters

This thrush has three thousand, three hundred and thirty-three feathers.

Tie the things that you have together with some string.

With these thoughts the author ends his thesis.

Are these sacks things that you want?

These three thrushes have fine, thick, silky feathers.

Tie the things you have together with this string.

The bathroom, thankfully, had three toothbrushes.

The oath is nothing to be enthralled or theatrical about.

Theoretically, the other author is more uncouth, but more wealthy.

The uncouth, but wealthy author had threadbare thermals.

S – Multisyllabic Words

sacrosanct	sagacious
salsify	saintliness
sanctimonious	saracen
soreness	somniferous
saturate	subsection
sesame	sinister
simultaneous	supersonic

Z – **Multisyllabic Words**

zealousness	zeppelin
zenithal	zincographer
zodiacal	zoography
zymotic	zophytic

S and Z – Tongue-Twisters

Sister Suzy sang us some sweet Sicilian songs.

Snip off those silly little bits with these scissors.

Sam collects horse-brasses and all sorts of glasses.

Some sailors suffer from seasickness.

The sinister servant said, 'Sir, supper is served.'

The messenger sat silently saying not a single word.

The dissatisfied assistant assassinated his master, the president.

I suppose the zebra is certainly nothing to lose sleep over.

Silvia understood from Simon, that Sonia was stopping selling cheese.

The house had a maze for those silly enough to be teased.

SC/SK

Initial	Medial	Final
sky	askew	ask
skill	disco	flask
scare	biscuit	desk
scam	escape	tusk
skin	basket	task
scone	Eskimo	mask
skater	descale	mosque
scales	telescope	rusk

Handout
92

scallywag	telescopically
scandalous	scarification
escarpment	scepticism
schizophrenia	sculptress
masquerade	skywriter
scholastic	scaffolding

SCR

scram	scrabble
scrap	scribble
scrape	scrimmage
scrawl	scratchy
scrimp	scripture
screen	scrutiny
screw	scrofula
script	scrapbook

SQU/SKW

squeak	squirrel
square	squiggle
squat	squabble
squaw	squirm
squirt	squeamish
squeeze	squeegee
squint	squarely
squib	squalor

Initial	*Medial*	*Final*
sly	coleslaw	n/a
slay	asleep	
sling	landslide	
slow	aslant	
slide		
slap		
sleeper		
slightly		

slapstick	slatternly
slaughterous	sleepiness
sleeveband	slipstream
slovenly	slow-worm
sloppiness	sliding-scale
slaughterhouse	slipshod

small	smaller
smell	smelly
smear	smoker
smirk	

SN

snap	snatch
sniff	snowman
snail	snooker
snare	snippet
snoop	snobbish

Initial	Medial	Final
spot	inspire	asp
spoon	espy	wasp
spat	aspire	wisp
spare	despite	rasp
spill	suspense	lisp
sparrow	dispense	cusp
speedy	despoil	
spatial	bespoke	

SP – Multisyllabic Words

spatula	spaghetti
speakable	speciality
specification	speciosity
spectacular	speculation
spellbound	spiritualist
spontaneously	spotlessly
bespectacled	suspensory

spray

sprout

sprig

sprint

spring

sprung

spread

spree

osprey

respray

bedspread

sprinkle

sprightly

sprocket

spreadable

sprinkling

Initial	Medial	Final
stop	tasty	oast
stem	misty	most
still	abstain	fast
stab	toaster	toast
steep	mustard	trust
stapler	thirsty	thirst
stagger	custard	burst
stable	asteroid	coast

Handout
102
© F Sugden-Best 2002

astonishment	stabilisation
stagnation	stage-whisper
astigmatism	stalactites
standardisation	consubstantiate
starvation	statistician
steadfastly	stenographer
steeplechase	astonishingly

Initial	Medial	Final
strike	restrain	n/a
stripe	restrict	
strap	restrung	
strain	unstrap	
struck	constrain	
stretch	construct	
straddle	construe	
struggle	outstretch	

STR – Multisyllabic Words

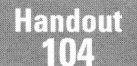

constrictive	straightforward
strategist	constructively
straitlaced	strenuously
strangulation	streptococcus
streptomycin	stringency
constringent	astringency
astrological	astrophysical

sway	sweater
sweat	swallow
switch	sweeper
swot	swelter
swan	swindler
sweet	swollen
swell	swivel
swop	swarthy

S plus consonants – Tongue-Twisters

Steven's swollen sweater made him swelter.

The straitlaced astrologist was struck by the strike.

Most toast, custard and mustard will make you thirsty.

The osprey sprang on to the spreadable bedspread.

The sparrow specifically liked wasps, asps and spaghetti.

Despite being bespectacled, he left them unspeakably spellbound.

The small snail was snobbish and smelly.

The slovenly slow-worm was asleep after the landslide.

The squid squirmed and squirted at the squinting squirrel.

He scrutinised the scribble in the scrawny scrapbook.

SH – Multisyllabic Words

shadowy	shamefully
shipshape	sharpshooter
shopwalker	showdown
shellshock	shoulderblade
shenanigan	shuttlecock
shovel hat	shortshrift
shock-absorber	shepherdess

SHR

shrug	shrapnel
shred	shrivel
shrill	shrinkage
shrive	shrunken
shrub	shrewdly
shroff	shrubbery
shrank	shrine
shrew	shrimps

SH – Tongue-Twisters

She showed me some machine-made horseshoes.

I wish to be shown the latest fashion in short skirts.

Mr Nash sells fresh shellfish from the seashore.

The sheep sheltered in a shed near a station.

He shaves his bushy moustache with short, sharp strokes.

He was shaking from the shock of being crushed in the rush.

He was ashamed of fishing for shrimps.

The shrubs were shaking from the shrew's shenanigans.

The shuttlecock was used as a shock-absorber by the shellshocked fisherman.

H – Tongue-Twisters

The happy hunter headed for the high hills.

The hunter hurriedly hid behind a high hedge.

The hard-hearted father disinherited his unhappy daughter.

He hailed him with a hearty hello and handshake.

The honey in hundreds of hives is heather honey.

Henry offered Hazel only half of his heart.

Hugh hurt his hand with a heavy hammer.

How do you harpoon a huge hippopatamus?

However you happen to help, Hugo has to hurry.

The horse's hoof was hurting horribly from the hammer.

J – Multisyllabic Words

jack-knife	January
jealously	jeopardise
jocularity	judicious
journalistc	juxtaposition
jujitsu	jurisdiction
justification	juggernaut
joviality	jocundity

CH – Multisyllabic Words

chairmanship	chalkiness
challenger	childishness
chambermaid	charitable
changeableness	churchwoman
chaffinch	chaplaincy
championship	chambermaid

*Sourcebook for Assessing &
Maintaining Communication*
© F Sugden-Best 2002

CH and J – Tongue-Twisters

Charles chose a cheap chop and chips for lunch.

The charming picture of a church in Chester was much admired.

Just for a joke, we mixed gin and ginger with Gerald's jam.

They chopped up the chains with a cheap chipped chopper.

He injured his thumb on the jagged edge of a broken jar.

The budgerigar and pigeon were jumping over the strange barge.

The pageboy fidgeted when the soldier just jumped.

The butcher chopped the chilli and chicken in the kitchen.

In January and July, badgers eat oranges and jelly in the orchard.

Y – Tongue-Twisters

Yesterday I heard a curious and beautiful new tune.

The beautiful music may make you yearn to hear more.

The youth told a peculiar yarn about a yellow yacht.

The yellowhammer yelled at you yesterday.

Yes, the yachtman's yacht is yet yours to borrow.

C/K – Multisyllabic Words

cacophony	calculate
caricature	cataract
catechism	compunction
communicable	cosmopolitan
corpulence	co-education
connective	confiscate
conversion	correspondence

CL/KL

Initial	*Medial*	*Final*
claw	nickles	chuckle
clean	tickles	nickle
class	tackles	
clap	pickles	
clip	cockles	
clop		
clinic		
clover		

CL/KL – Multisyllabic Words

clairaudience	clairvoyance
clamorously	clannishness
clarification	classification
clearing-station	cloistered
clumsiness	cleverness

cry	credulous
crowd	credentials
cried	crematorium
crew	crepitate
crawl	criterion
cravat	crocodile
craving	crucifixion
creepy	cryogenics

quack	quadruple
quake	quadruped
qualm	quarterstaff
quash	quarantine
quaver	questionable
queenly	quinquennial
quibble	quotation
quinine	quixotism

C and K – Tongue-Twisters

I acquired a quaint copper kettle in the market.

If we keep quiet, we may be lucky and see the cuckoo.

Uncle Kenneth's black cat Kim is quite an inquisitive creature.

The cream-coloured car collided with a cart.

Take care not to make mistakes when you bake those cakes.

The crowd cried for a cacophony of clarifications.

The donkey and cow hiked to the circus in Canada to co-star.

He calculated the cost of quarantining the lucky kipper.

The sulky hiker had a craving to crawl and claw to the clearing-station.

G – Multisyllabic Words

galligaskins	gainsay
gargantuan	galvanisation
gastronomical	gazetteer
galley-slave	galvanism
go-getter	goldsmith
guardianship	gynaecology
gondolier	gorgonzola
governmental	gumption

GL – Multisyllabic Words

glue	glengarry
glow	globular
glare	glycerine
gloat	glottalic
glaze	glyptograph
glacier	glossary
glider	glimmering
glimmer	glorification

Initial	Medial	Final
grey	angry	n/a
grade	agree	
great	regrade	
grim	regroup	
groan	peregrine	
gradual	telegram	
grammar	engrave	
griddle	milligram	

Handout
124
© F Sugden-Best 2002

upgradeable	greengrocery
gravitation	graminivorous
ingratiatingly	gramophone
grandiloquence	graduation
graciously	telegrammatic
grammatically	agricultural
agreeability	agreeableness

G – Tongue-Twisters

The great king gave guests magnificent gifts of gold.

If you go digging in the garden, wear your old grey gloves.

The good guide got all our gear together.

The grey geese gave angry warnings when the hungry wolf came.

The alligator was greyish-brown with a great big mouth.

The great peregrine glided close to the glimmering glacier.

He guarded the grateful girl who was going to Greenland.

The tiger wore a saggy toga, given by the greengrocer.

NG – Multisyllabic Words

boomerang	languidly
languorous	lengthily
linguistic	longanimity
longshoreman	longitudinal
singlestick	dungarees
ringleader	pangolin

NG – Tongue-Twisters

Bring those things in and hand them over.

Uncle hurt his ankle at the ice-skating rink.

I think she lost her ring in the throng at the banquet.

The spring brings many charming things.

Mr King was playing and singing a rousing song.

He lingered, longing for the band to play a tango.

Running, walking and singing are all things that a king can do.

The stronger the pungency, the longer the smell lingers.

The boomerang banged into the long tongue of the ringleader.

Two-Syllable Words

headache	kitten
wheelchair	today
upset	happen
happy	apple
doctor	bottle
mother	toilet
outside	tissue
inside	pencil
dinner	repeat

Three-Syllable Words

hospital	insulin
charity	injection
relative	confident
criticise	unhelpful
appetite	argument
pyjamas	overcoat
computer	library
consultant	understand
aggravate	bandages

Four-Syllable Words

thermometer	confidential
experienced	therapeutic
sympathetic	invisible
ventilation	aggravation
ridiculous	unhappily
accountable	unhygienic
understatement	violation
regrettable	benefactor
superstitious	rediscover

astronomical	understandably
anniversary	radiographer
legibility	alphabetical
unacceptable	accommodation
pharmaceutical	amplification
miscellaneous	defribrillation
masculinity	liability
procrastination	undeniably
unrepeatable	recommendation

Six-Syllable Words

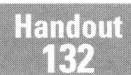

respectability

unsympathetically

humanitarian

identification

juxtapositional

impossibility

decontamination

unexceptionally

authoritarian

deterioration

idiosyncracy

respectability

prioritisation

unequivocally

encyclopaedia

nationalisation

potentiality

interrogatory

Three-Syllable Sentences

What's the time?	It is late.
How are you?	Where is Sue?
It's a dog.	Fires are warm.
Time for tea.	Snow is cold.
Where's my bed?	Wool is light.
Who are you?	Gym is fun.
I am sad.	Close the door.
I like red.	Pigeons fly.
Tim is fast.	Turtles swim.

Four-Syllable Sentences

Is it your turn?

Salads are cold.

Tom is hungry.

Crisps are crunchy.

Trousers are warm.

Winter is cold.

Rabbits run fast.

Hares run quicker.

Where has Jim gone?

John is heavy.

Open the door.

I like kittens.

Where is the sun?

It is July.

Worms are slimy.

How old are you?

Is it three yet?

I am happy.

Five-Syllable Sentences

Say that again please.

Make a cup of tea

Time to go away.

How long does it take?

Geoffrey is playing.

Is this seat taken?

Alfred is clever.

The dustbin is full.

Cabbages are green.

Six-Syllable Sentences

Julian is fasting.

Jessica is crying.

Give the dog a biscuit.

Hide under the table.

Go outside the door now.

Let's take a drive to France.

The twins are three years old.

She loves chocolate cake.

Have you been to Paris?

Seven-Syllable Sentences

Where is the one you wanted?

Jeremy and Bill are friends.

Did you enjoy the new play?

Have you been to Madeira?

Is it two twenty-five yet?

Susan is big for her age.

Tadpoles grow into small frogs.

Sid sent Sue some big flowers.

Do you like dogs or cats best?

Multisyllabic Sentences

The radioactive isotope could cause a catastrophic explosion.

Surprisingly, the uncommunicative man was a psychoanalyst.

For rehabilitation to be effective, one must identify the seemingly insurmountable obstacles.

For clarification on numerical calculations, consult the mathematician.

The encyclopaedia is prioritised alphabetically as recommended by the publisher.

Understandably the professional consultant was unconsolable.

Chapter 4

Communication Handouts

This chapter contains a selection of communication handouts, which have been designed for clinicians to give out to anyone – for example, a relative, carer or nurse who needs to communicate with someone who experiences problems participating fully in a communication situation. It may be that the people with the communication impairment could also benefit from being given some of the sheets themselves; so with this in mind, the font and sizing have been chosen to aid visual acuity. Several of the handouts may be appropriate to be given out as a set – for example, the stroke patient over 65, who is hard of hearing and has right-sided facial weakness, may benefit from the sheets on dysarthria, hearing impairment and communicating with the elderly person.

The sheets cover the following subjects:

◆ What is communication?
◆ What are the effects of normal ageing on communication?
◆ Strategies for communicating with an elderly person
◆ Strategies for communicating with the hard of hearing
◆ Communicating with the hearing-aid wearer
◆ The listener in communication situations
◆ The speaker in communication situations
◆ What is dysphasia?
◆ What is dysarthria?
◆ What is dementia?
◆ Strategies for communicating with a dysphasic partner
◆ Strategies for communicating with a dysarthric partner

What is Communication?

Name _____ Date _____

Normal communication is a combination of both verbal and non-verbal means of expression. Communication, therefore, can involve one or all of the following during an interaction:

Appearance   How we interact with someone depends on how they appear to us – for example, a vagrant versus our favourite film star.

Eye contact   Communication is difficult when we are unable to gain eye contact with someone.

Facial expression   We use our faces to show how we are feeling.

Touch   We can touch someone to gain attention; some cultures use touch more than others.

Crying/Laughter   These are extreme emotions, which demonstrate how sad or happy we are.

Gesture   For example, we point to show where something is, or wave to say 'hello or goodbye'.

Listening   We have to listen to someone we are communicating with in order to reply appropriately.

Tone of voice   If we are bored, our voices sound bored. News readers do not reveal how they personally feel as they report on tragic events.

Speech/Writing   Sometimes we need to communicate by writing, such as sending a letter; sometimes by talking.

Effective communication involves two or more people – the speaker(s) and listener(s) – both following the verbal language and non-verbal signs.

The main aim of communication is to transfer information, and the key to this process is listening.

What are the Effects of Normal Ageing on Communication?

Name _____ Date _____

This handout is designed to help you understand the effect that normal ageing can have on communication, and to highlight why elderly people need additional support from the listener in a conversation.

Hearing

◆ If there is a reduction in the ability to hear, there may be difficulties with hearing and therefore understanding speech.

◆ If there are hearing problems, comprehension can be difficult if the person is spoken to quickly.

Vision

◆ If there is impairment in vision due to, for example, clouding and/or pathological changes such as glaucoma, the result is a reduction in acuity and focusing power, and problems with colour discrimination.

◆ If there are visual problems, the person requires a longer period of time to look at material, and needs encouragement to scan – that is to look at – everything in front of them.

◆ Material needs to be shown much more slowly if there is a visual problem.

Motor slowing

◆ Reaction time, or the person's ability to respond, may slow down if there are distractions, such as the radio being on, or if the person is tired.

◆ Factors such as familiarity with the stimulus – for example, a picture of a close family member seen regularly when compared to one of a distant cousin usually seen only once a year – may affect interaction.

What are the Effects of Normal Ageing on Communication? *...continued*

Memory

◆ The person may have difficulty retaining more recent information, such as what they did the day before.

◆ The person may be slow at retrieving information from the long-term memory – that is, things that happened a little while ago.

Attention/Concentration

◆ The person may have difficulty attending to difficult or complex activities, particularly if complicated instructions, either written or spoken, are given.

◆ It may be difficult for the person to multi-task – that is, to do several things at the same time – for example, watch television, eat a meal and talk to a friend.

◆ The person may have difficulty bringing together lots of different pieces of information, and be unable to ignore irrelevant or distracting pieces of information – for example, drawing together a newspaper story.

◆ The person may need someone else to help – for example, to turn the television off when they are reading to aid attention/concentration, rather than thinking of doing it independently.

Language/Understanding

◆ The person's understanding will usually remain intact in relation to their own individual environment.

◆ There may be difficulty comprehending complicated language, but words and simple sentences are usually understood with no difficulty.

◆ The person may have difficulty with the following:

1 Being spoken to at a fast rate

2 Having to concentrate on lots of things at once

3 Remembering what they are doing, because activities take longer to complete

4 If there are hearing and/or visual problems, it can be easy to miss non-verbal cues, such as, facial expression.

Psychosocial

◆ The person's own self-concept of what it feels like to be elderly; their individual personality, and society's concept of the older person will affect the ageing process.

◆ If the person has poor motivation, this will reduce performance.

◆ The person may not want to 'take on board' new information, or learn new skills.

◆ The person may fatigue more easily.

◆ There is more ill health in the elderly population, with an increase in multiple incidences of illness rather than isolated problems.

◆ Depression is more prevalent in the elderly.

Sociocultural

◆ Elderly people may present differently depending on whether they are in their own home or an institution.

◆ Cultural perspectives of roles in life and/or status may change with growing old age.

◆ Expectations may cause problems – for example, cooperation and motivation could be affected if the person has not been faced with the prospect of having speech and language therapy before.

◆ The person may be anxious, and this may be especially related to fear of failure.

It is important to note that an older person may not perform as well on intelligence tasks due to the reduced speed of performance in reaction times and decreased processing ability (that is, slowing of motor movement and ability to respond quickly to questions). Therefore, it may not be intelligence *per se* that changes with age.

Strategies for Communicating with an Elderly Person

Name _____ Date _____

This handout is designed to remind you of the things you need to consider when communicating with someone who is elderly.

1 Make sure the person is wearing glasses, hearing aid(s) and dentures, if required.

2 Do not speak 'down' to the person, treat them as you yourself would wish to be treated. Older does not mean less adult or less quick-witted.

3 Allow the person time to understand, to reply and to accept new faces and change.

4 Make sure you give the person the chance to direct the conversation, participating as fully as any adult would.

5 If the person has difficulty understanding, repeat new information as often as is necessary to give adequate time to adjust.

6 Do not change topics quickly in conversation.

7 Do not expect the person to concentrate for very long.

8 If you are unsure whether the person has understood, ask them to repeat what you have just said, or say it more slowly. Demonstrate what you would like them to do.

9 Allow the person time to talk about what is important to them, no matter how trivial it may appear to you.

10 Allow the person time to talk about what is troubling them, especially about death.

11 People age at different rates, so do not assume that just because a person is 90 years old, their ability to hold a conversation will be impaired. Do not judge an Ondividual by chronological age. Each individual will have different abilities.

Strategies for Communicating with the Hard of Hearing

Name _____ Date _____

This handout is designed to remind you of the things to consider when communicating with someone who is hard of hearing.

1 If the person has a hearing aid, make sure it is in the correct ear and working properly (see separate sheet on hearing aids). Make sure they are wearing glasses, dentures, etc, if required.

2 Make sure the surroundings are as quiet as possible. Turn down the radio/television, close doors/windows if there is noise outside.

3 Let the light fall on your face so the person can see your lips, facial expression and gesture.

4 Avoid gestures and hand movements that cover your mouth.

5 Do not speak while chewing or eating.

6 Before speaking, gain attention by, for example, touching the shoulder. If the person is in a chair, bend or sit down so your faces are at the same level.

7 Speak clearly and slowly, without exaggerating your mouth movements. Do not shout, but speak at a good, loud level.

8 If you know the person can hear better on one side than the other, speak to that side.

9 If you are in a group, give the person a clue as to what you are talking about, avoiding sudden changes in topic.

10 Avoid long, involved sentences. If repetition is required, rephrase the sentence to make it shorter and simpler. Do not talk 'down' to the person with a hearing impairment.

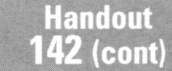

Strategies for Communicating with the Hard of Hearing ...*continued*

11 Use signs or pointing to illustrate, if appropriate.

12 Do not forget the person may find communicating easier if you write everything down, or use 'key' words.

13 If telling a complex story, check at regular intervals to see if the person is following.

14 Be conscious that some people are embarrassed by their hearing difficulty, so indicate that you understand and are willing to help.

Communicating with the Hearing-Aid Wearer

Name _____ Date _____

This handout is designed to remind you of the things to consider when communicating with someone who wears a hearing aid.

1 Encourage the user to wear their hearing aid(s) all the time.

2 Make sure you know how the aid works. Know how to change batteries and set the volume control appropriately.

3 Encourage prompt attendance at the appropriate clinic if the aid is not working properly, or contact the clinic for advice.

4 Encourage the user to attend for regular check-ups, as the aid(s) may need updating.

The Listener in Communication Situations

Name _____ Date _____

This handout is designed to remind you how to help the speech-impaired person in a communication situation.

1　It is the role of the listener to modify the physical environment of the communicatively impaired person by:

◆ Reducing sources of noise and increasing the opportunity for the speaker to hear the listener – for example, turning the television or radio off or down, and having rugs on wooden floors

◆ Avoiding noisy and dark settings

◆ Maintaining eye contact

◆ Maintaining direct face-to-face contact

◆ Limiting your distance from the speaker.

2　The listener needs to maximise their own hearing and visual acuity by wearing hearing aid(s) and glasses.

3　The listener needs to actively listen by:

◆ Giving the speaker full attention

◆ Checking constantly with the speaker that they are understanding

◆ Letting the speaker know as soon as possible when they have not understood.

The Speaker in Communication Situations

Name _____ Date _____

This handout is designed to help you manage communication situations effectively.

Managing your surroundings

1 If possible, eliminate background noise – for example, by turning down the radio, or moving to quieter surroundings.

2 Try to move closer to your listener or get them to move close to you. Make sure you can see each other's faces.

3 If the listener is wearing a hearing aid, check that it is working.

Before you speak

1 Think in advance what you are going to say, and try to keep it short and concise.

2 Face your listener and check that they are watching and attending to you before you speak.

3 Attract the listener to the fact that you wish to communicate by touch, calling their name, making some sound.

As you speak

1 Always speak slowly, articulating words as clearly as possible. Use your full range of lip and tongue movements.

2 Make speech as precise as possible, exaggerating the articulation if necessary.

3 Try not to say too much on one breath. If your voice is fading, it could be a sign that you need to take in more air, so stop and start again.

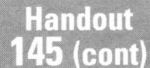
The Speaker in Communication Situations ...continued

4 Encourage others to turn off the television or radio and shut windows and doors, so it is easier for the listener to hear your speech.

5 To stop the words from running together, pause frequently, giving extra time to take extra breaths.

6 Practise any oral and/or breathing exercises you have been given regularly, to help maintain your current ability and strengthen the facial muscles, especially those used for speech.

7 Practise problem words and phrases.

8 Remember the ends of words.

9 Sound every SYL – LA – BLE.

What is Dysphasia?

Name _____ Date _____

Dysphasia is a specific impairment of language, which can affect all aspects of communication. It results in total or partial impairment of the ability to formulate, express or understand the meaning of spoken and/or written words.

It is due to an isolated (focal) lesion in the dominant (ie, left) cerebral hemisphere, resulting from a stroke (CVA).

In addition, there may be difficulty in reading (dyslexia) and writing (dysgraphia), and failure to understand gestures and signs (asymbolia) or music (amusia).

A person with dysphasia – that is a breakdown in language – will have difficulties in varying degrees in some or all four areas of language:

1 Auditory comprehension   – the understanding of spoken language

2 Reading comprehension   – the understanding of written language

3 Verbal expression   – speech

4 Written expression   – writing

What is Dysarthria?

Name _____ Date _____

Dysarthria is the name given to the group of speech disorders that result in difficulty controlling the muscular movements of the speech mechanism – that is, the lips, tongue, palate, larynx and breathing.

This is due to nerve damage, either on one side (unilateral) – as may occur in the event of a single stroke – or both sides (bilateral) – as in some progressive neurological conditions.

The person's speech becomes slurred (imprecise) and slows down. The tone can become monotonous, and dribbling may occur from the side of the mouth if there is lip weakness.

Causes of dysarthria include:

◆ Stroke (CVA)

◆ Multiple sclerosis

◆ Head injury

◆ Parkinson's disease

◆ Motor Neurone disease

◆ Huntington's disease

◆ Friedreich's ataxia.

What is Dementia?

Handout
148

Name _____ Date _____

Dementia occurs more commonly in older people, resulting in the deterioration of intellectual functions, so there can be impairment of memory, intelligence and a wide variety of aptitudes and accomplishments.

Dementia can affect speech. For example, names of objects may be inaccurate, and speech may be simplified, consisting only of statements, descriptions or requests of little or no importance. There may be failure to comprehend verbal instructions and follow conversation, resulting in complete communication breakdown.

Strategies for Communicating with a Dysphasic Partner – Sheet 1

Name _____ Date _____

This handout is designed to remind you of things to consider when communicating with someone who has dysphasia.

1 Make sure you are speaking face-to-face with the person. If necessary, bend or sit down so you are at the same eye level. Do not address the person from behind, or turn away as you are communicating with them.

2 Cue the person – for example, touch their arm, smile, make some pleasant general remarks or comments, use their name before launching into a conversation. Do not start the conversation with complex questions or comments without warning.

3 Talk in a quiet, relaxed environment, free from distractions.

4 Ensure only one person is communicating with the dysphasic person at a time.

5 Make sure the person has a clear means of indicating yes and no so that basic questions, such as 'Would you like a cup of coffee?', can be answered easily. Open-ended questions can be more difficult to answer – that is, those beginning with who, what, where, when, why and how.

6 As the listener, you may need to carry the burden of the conversation. Do not limit the conversation to questions, but spend time reassuring and telling the person what is going on.

7 Do speak simply and slowly, but do not 'talk down' to the person. Many people with dysphasia feel they are losing their minds, which could be reinforced if someone is patronising.

8 Do give the person plenty of time to understand, consider and respond. They may require more time due to slowing of the thought processes. Do not rush on to the next topic, particularly if you have posed a question.

9 Do make every effort to interpret the person's needs and views, but don't ever pretend to understand the person when you do not.

10 Give the person your undivided attention when they are speaking. Do not think about other things – that is, half listen – otherwise you may miss the opportunity to ask questions to clarify the intended message.

11 Be prepared to repeat your comments or questions, but try not to raise your voice unnecessarily.

12 Be specific with questions or remarks, emphasising key words and placing pauses before important words in sentences. Do not ramble – for example, 'I'm not sure exactly what time your daughter said she would be here, was it 2.00 pm or 4.00 pm, but I'm sure you would be free for an eye appointment at 2.30 pm. What do you think?'

13 Encourage automatic speech, as it is often easy for the person to use social greetings and exchanges, for example, 'Hello', 'How are you?' This can help to prompt feelings of adequacy in a communicative environment.

14 Use lively, appropriate facial expression, even if it feels slightly exaggerated – for example, frowning to emphasise sadness, smiling for good news. Do not speak with an expressionless face, as it could be interpreted as boredom or disapproval.

15 Do not 'correct' errors; encourage but do not pressurise further responses.

16 Encourage the person to communicate in any way possible, including gesture, writing, etc. Do not insist on the person using speech if other ways enable them to communicate more easily. Communication, not speech, is the important factor.

Strategies for Communicating with a Dysphasic Partner – Sheet 1 ...continued

17 Do not be surprised, upset or show amusement if the person swears more than they are used to, as swearing can be common following a stroke. Provide the correct word without showing emotion. Try not to show embarrassment if the person cries easily; maintain communication in a matter of fact way. These extremes of emotions may be very embarrassing and upsetting for the person too.

18 Avoid talking for the person as words you use may not be what they intended to say.

19 Avoid abstract and vague topics.

20 Make every opportunity to engage in conversation, to provide stimulation to talk about topics of interest to them.

21 Ability may fluctuate, so some days will be better than others for individuals as regards finding the right words.

22 Never talk about the person in their presence as though they were not there, as no matter how severe the comprehension problems, the person may be able to grasp limited bits of information that could be distressing.

Strategies for Communicating with a Dysphasic Partner – Sheet 2

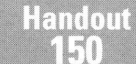

Name _____ Date _____

This handout is designed to be a quick reminder of strategies to use when communicating with a dysphasic speaking partner.

Slow down your speech rate

◆ Slow down your overall speech rate.

◆ If you are introducing a difficult or important topic or repeating/ rephrasing a sentence that has been misunderstood by the listener, slow down even more.

Pausing

◆ Break a longer sentence into ideas or chunks, using pausing.

◆ Within a sentence, say words slowly and clearly.

◆ Allow a pause between two consecutive sentences, by silently counting to five at the end of the first sentence, before continuing.

◆ If you are expecting an answer or response from the listener, allow a five-second pause after finishing the sentence, to give time for them to formulate an idea and begin to speak.

◆ Sometimes it may be necessary to wait for up to 12 seconds before a response is given.

Use straightforward sentences

◆ Specify who, what, where and when. For example:

'I was watching it last night.'   'I was watching Eastenders last night.'

'She came yesterday.'   'Julia came yesterday.'

'John went there last summer.'   'John went to France last summer.'

Strategies for Communicating with a Dysphasic Partner – Sheet 2 ...continued

Changing topic

◆ Change your general body posture by leaning forward, for example, to introduce a new topic.

◆ Use a gesture to close a topic – for example, close your hands together.

◆ Terminate the topic with a statement – for example, 'I should be going now.'

◆ Use an introductory statement for new topics – for example, 'Have you heard about?'

◆ Use a pause of at least five seconds between topics.

◆ Repeat the subject or key words of the topic – for example, 'Shall we have burgers tonight? Should I buy burgers in Sainsbury's for tonight?'

Use alerters

◆ When starting a conversation, do not begin with the important items, but instead give time for the person to tune in and listen to you.

◆ Touch the person and pause before speaking.

◆ Use the person's name before starting a conversation.

◆ Use a verbal lead-in, for example, 'What do you think about?' 'By the way'.

Strategies for Communicating with a Dysarthric Partner

Name _____ Date _____

This handout is designed to remind you of the things you need to consider when communicating with someone with dysarthria.

1 The more you know the person, the more familiar you will be with their speech, and the easier it will be for you to understand the person. Therefore, the more you talk to the person, the more familiar you will become with their speech and the easier it will be for you to understand.

2 Check that hearing aid(s), glasses and dentures, if required, are in place and check that they are 'fit for use'.

3 Face the speaker so you can watch their mouth, as watching the person's lips will often aid understanding.

4 Make the surroundings as quiet as possible, by turning off the television or radio, and shutting doors and windows.

5 Do not speak at the same time, or interrupt.

6 There is no need to raise your voice unless the person has a hearing problem.

7 Do not get agitated, if you are not understanding; be patient and tolerant. Stay calm because agitation will stop you from listening and further agitate the speaker. The person's speech will be slow and effortful, so remind them that you will leave them enough time.

8 Ask the speaker to spell out particular words you are having difficulty with.

9 Ask for a repetition if you are unsure as to whether you have understood. Ask the person to repeat one word at a time if necessary, and say each word back to confirm that you have understood. Indicate to the person if they are speaking too quickly for you to understand.

Strategies for Communicating with a Dysarthric
Partner ...*continued*

10 Ask questions requiring only a yes/no response to define the context of the conversation if you are not understanding.

11 During conversation, repeat the part of the message you can understand. Ask appropriate questions to establish the message if you are having difficulty. Nodding also shows that you are following what the person is saying.

12 Ask the person to repeat the key word or words in the conversation as this will help you to understand.

13 Never pretend to understand the person when you don't. It will often be obvious to the speaker that you have not understood, which will result in greater frustration.

14 Ask the person if there is any way that they can show you or take you somewhere to make the subject matter clearer.

15 Tell the speaker as soon as you are experiencing problems understanding. Otherwise there is potential for large amounts of information to be lost.

16 If possible, encourage all attempts at speech, but if the person is able physically to write or point to a communication chart, use these methods to supplement/complement speech.

17 Sometimes a person with dysarthria will also have cognitive and/or expressive language difficulties, so that what they say may not be appropriate, thus making it more difficult to understand.

18 If you cannot understand, and time is limited, ask the person if it is important or if it can wait until a later time. If it is important, perhaps somebody else may be available to assist you.

Chapter 5

Assessment of Communication Skills

This chapter comprises a set of screens:

1   **Initial language screen.** This screen is designed to be used at the bedside, to give an overall impression of language function in all modalities. Administration sheets are included for many of the sub-sections; these can be cut up and laminated, or covered in sticky-backed plastic. Some sheets have a range of choices, so please take into account the use of semantically related words, and also the potential for confusion with nouns that become verbs – for example, 'comb to combing' for some individuals. Clinicians can take their own stimulation pictures and use items from around the bedside or familiar objects for the remaining sub-sections, or if they feel the words and stimuli suggested are not appropriate. For the colour-matching screen, the triangles on the photocopiable masters contain the name of the appropriate colour, with colour samples in the Appendixes.

The client could also write or talk about an important or recent event in the written expression/picture description sections. The score sheet is small, but this allows the results to be contained on one page as a summary sheet.

2   **Screen of linguistic concepts.** This screen is designed to test the client's ability to comprehend complex sentences, while assessing five linguistic concepts.

Each of the five sections has a separate presentation sheet, with a score sheet. The subject either points directly with a hand, or eye points to their choice. It may help to score 0.5 if the person achieves the task, but chooses in the wrong order, on some of the sub-sections.

The five sections are:
◆ Inclusion/Exclusion (not, except, all but one, either)
◆ Temporal (after, before)
◆ Conditional (instead of, if, until, when)
◆ Coordination (and)
◆ Quantitative (all, some, any one, all but one, first)

Once again colour is indicated on the blank masters to copy and colour, and colour samples are provided in the Appendixes.

3 **Dysphasia/Dementia screen.** This form is a useful guide to the main differences between the two conditions, although it should be stressed that there will be considerable individual variation.

Initial Language Screen

Name _____ Date _____

DOB _____ Diagnosis _____ _____

Handedness   Right   Left   First language _____

Visual impairment _____

Hearing impairment _____

Physical impairment _____

Visual matching

1	Colour to colour	/4
2	Shape to shape	/4
3	Letter to letter	/4
4	Number to number	/4
5	Object to object	/4
6	Object to picture	/4
7	Object to gesture	/4
8	Picture to gesture	/4

(If the client does not have the motor ability, then use eye pointing or allow Yes/No choice on each question.)

Orientation *(Note Yes/No confusion)*

Are you in hospital?	Y/N	Are you at home?	Y/N	PLACE	Y/N
Is your name (wrong)?	Y/N	Is your name (correct)?	Y/N	PERSON	Y/N
Is the month/year (correct)?	Y/N	Is the month/year (wrong)?	Y/N	TIME	Y/N

/3

Auditory comprehension

1	Object to spoken word	/4
2	Picture to spoken word	/4
3	Picture (verb) to spoken word	/4
4	Object to function	/4
5	One-part commands Touch the comb. Touch the glass. Touch the tissue. Touch the spoon.	

(Note attention/concentration/distractibility/ behaviour/awareness.)

(Objects required are pen, glass, comb, spoon and tissue. Instruct that you will be asking them to touch or look at objects.)

/4

Initial Language Screen   ...continued

6a Two-part commands/questions
Touch the pen and comb.
Touch the tissue and glass.
Is rain wet?
Are elephants small?   /4

6b Left/right discrimination
Touch your left leg.
Touch your right ear.
Touch your right arm.
Touch your left knee.   /4

7 Three part commands/questions   *(Note whether carried out in the correct order.)*
Touch the tissue before the glass.
Do you dry yourself before a bath?
Touch the spoon, pen and comb.
Are daffodils and tomatoes both flowers?   /4

8 Four-part commands/questions
Do both cats and computers have fur?
Touch the pen and comb before the glass.
Are leopards, cheetahs and tigers all of the cat family?
Is Blackpool the biggest city in the world?   /4

Reasoning

Bill is older than Bob. Is Bob younger?	Y/N	
I want to lose weight. Should I eat more?	Y/N	
Is an elephant heavier than a mouse?	Y/N	
Sam is happier than Jan. Is Jan happiest?	Y/N	/4

Reading comprehension

1 Letters – D H B W   /4
2 Numbers – 4 11 9 30   /4
3 Object to word   /4
4 Picture to word   /4
5 Object to word (verb)   /4
6 Picture to word (verb)   /4
7 Sentence to picture   /4

Initial Language Screen   *...continued*

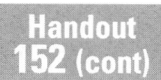

8   One-part commands
Touch the tissue.
Touch the glass.
Touch the spoon.
Touch the pen.

(Objects required are spoon, glass, pen, comb and tissue.)

/4

9a   Two-part commands/questions
Touch the pen and spoon.
Touch the glass and comb.
Do dogs fly?
Is water wet?

(Note whether carried out in the correct order.)

/4

9b   Left/right discrimination
Touch your left cheek.
Touch your right knee.
Touch your right ear.
Touch your left elbow.

/4

10   Three-part commands/questions
Touch the spoon before the glass.
Touch the pen, tissue and comb.
Do mice have long tails?
Do teachers work in banks?

/4

11   Four-part commands/questions
Touch the pen and comb after the spoon.
Is a kitten bigger than a fully grown cat?
Do fish and dogs both live in the sea?
Do you buy pills and deodorant in a chemist?

/4

Spoken expression

1   Name body parts

(Note use of gesture and alternative/ augmentative means of communication.)

Eye	Semantic cue:	Used to see with.
	Phonemic cue:	Begins with the sound E__
Nose	Semantic cue:	It needs a blow when you have a cold.
	Phonemic cue:	Begins with ...
Hand	Semantic cue:	You can wear gloves on these.
	Phonemic cue:	Begins with ...
Foot	Semantic cue:	You can wear shoes on these.
	Phonemic cue:	Begins with ...

/4

Initial Language Screen ...*continued*

2 Name objects

Bed	Semantic cue:	Used to sleep in.
	Phonemic cue:	Begins with …
Chair	Semantic cue:	Used to sit in.
	Phonemic cue:	Begins with …
Glass	Semantic cue:	Used to drink from.
	Phonemic cue:	Begins with …
Pen	Semantic cue:	Used to write with.
	Phonemic cue:	Begins with …

/4

3 Verb usage   Sleeping   Sitting
              Drinking   Writing

/4

4 Spontaneous expression
(name and address)

/4

5 Sentence completion
Wash your _____
A slice of _____
In _____ it can snow.
You buy _____ in a supermarket.

/4

6 Picture description *or* short story/recent event
(Use a separate sheet to record information.)

/4

Written expression

1 Copying (letters) – A G E X   /4
Recall (look then write letter by letter) – D J Y H   /4
Dictation – F B T C   /4

2 Copying (numbers) – 4 12 6 34   /4
Recall (number by number) – 5 10 7 8   /4
Dictation – 20 7 3 56   /4

3 Copying (words) – dog back drummer wardrobe   /4
Recall (words) – box help rain pillow   /4
Dictation – hot   _____
          – test   _____
          – object   _____
          – telephone   _____   /4

Handout
152 (cont)
© F Sugden-Best 2002

4 Sentence dictation
The man is running.
The door is open.
What is the time?
It is time for dinner. /4

5 Written object names – pen _____
          – chair _____
          – glass _____
          – watch _____ /4

6 Object usage – writing _____
          – sitting _____
          – drinking _____
          – telling the time _____ /4

7 Sentence completion
A loaf of _____.
Children enjoy going to the _____.
People go to the cinema to watch a _____.
When it is cold you _____ the door /4

8a Sentence construction
Write short sentences using one of the following words in each:
house
school
walking
drinking /4

8b Write a sentence using the following words
(a) In any order:
    house, cat, children
    food, work, late

(b) In order specified;
    summertime, barbecue, garden
    winter, early, lights /4

9 Spontaneous writing
(name and address)

/4

10 Picture description or short story/recent event.
(Use a separate sheet to record information.) /4

Initial Language Screen Results Sheet

Name _____ Date _____

SECTION	SCORE	COMMENTS
VISUAL MATCHING	Colour to colour Shape to shape Letter to letter Number to number Object to object Object to picture Object to gesture Picture to gesture TOTAL /32	
ORIENTATION	Place/Person/Time TOTAL /3	
AUDITORY COMPREHENSION	Object to spoken word Picture to spoken word Picture (verb) to spoken word Object to function One-part commands Two-part commands/questions Left/right discrimination Three-part commands/questions Four-part commands/questions TOTAL /36	
REASONING	TOTAL /4	
READING COMPREHENSION	Letter to letter Number to number Object to word Picture to word Object to word (verb) Picture to word (verb) Sentence to picture One-part commands Two-part commands/questions Left/right discrimination Three-part commands/questions Four-part commands/questions TOTAL /48	

Initial Language Screen Results Sheet *...continued*

SECTION	SCORE	COMMENTS
SPOKEN EXPRESSION	Body parts (semantic/phonemic cueing – Yes/No) Objects (semantic/phonemic cueing – Yes/No) Verb usage Spontaneous expression Sentence completion Picture description/short story TOTAL /24	
WRITTEN EXPRESSION	Copying letters Letter recall Letter dictation Copying numbers Number recall Number dictation Copying words Word recall Word dictation Sentence dictation Object naming Object usage Sentence completion Sentence construction Spontaneous writing Picture description/short story TOTAL /64	

Handout 154

Initial Language Screen: Visual Matching 1 – Colour to Colour

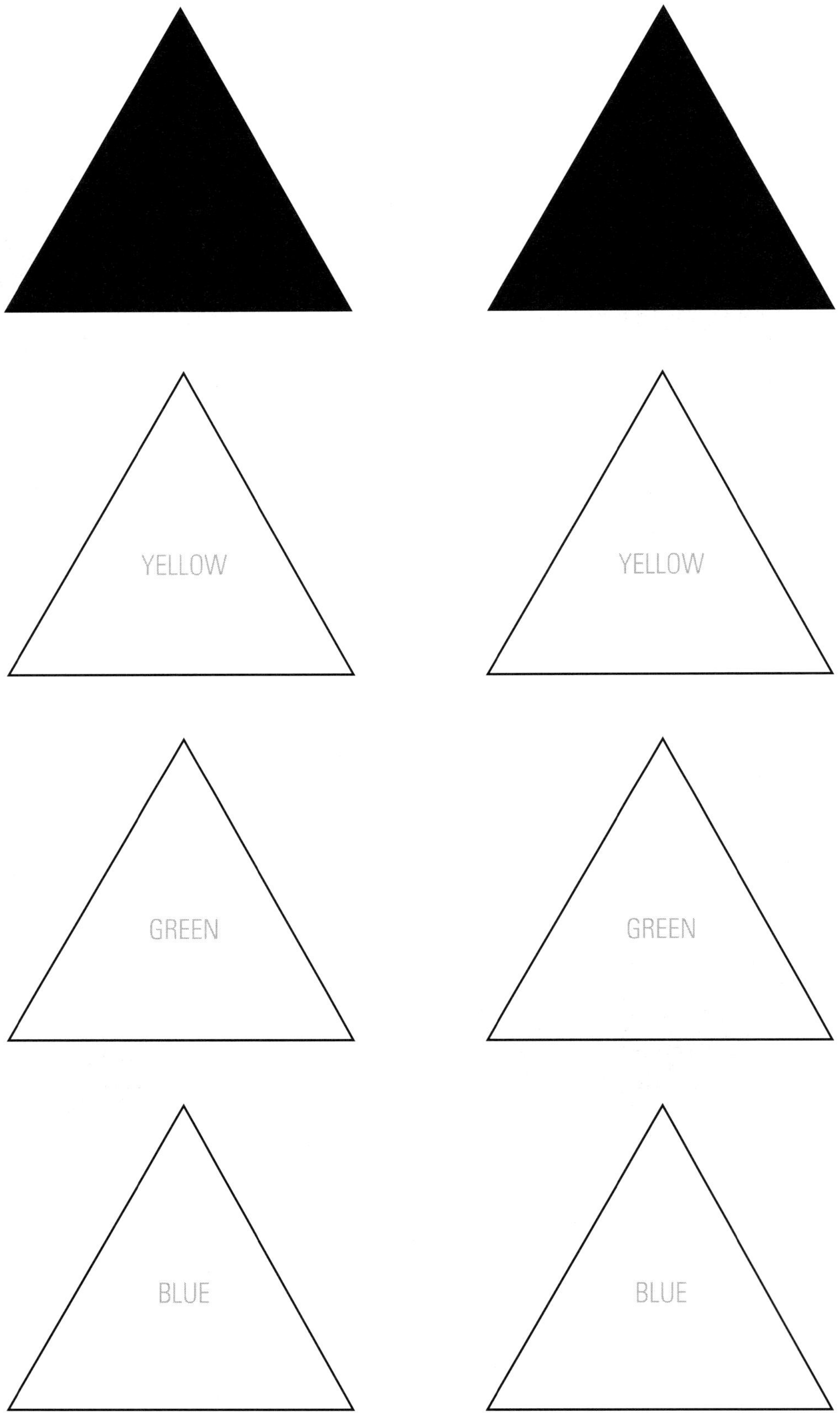
YELLOW
YELLOW
GREEN
GREEN
BLUE
BLUE

Initial Language Screen: Visual Matching 2 – Shape to Shape

Handout
155

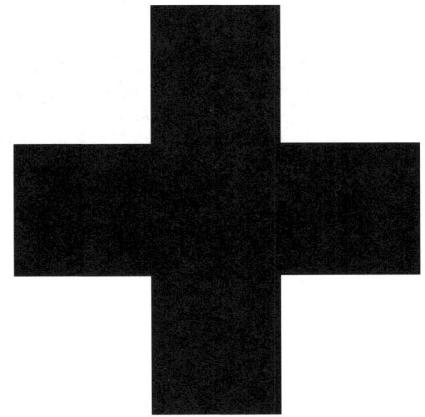

B O

K R

5   8

20 16

Initial Language Screen:
Reading Comprehension

(Uncover each section in isolation)

1 Letters

D H B W

2 Numbers

4 11 9 30

3 and **4**   Object/Picture to word

glass   spoon

comb   tissue

5 and **6** Reading verbs (object/picture) choices

sleeping   writing

sitting   drinking

eating   brushing

combing   washing

7 One-part commands

Touch the tissue.

Touch the glass.

Touch the spoon.

Touch the pen.

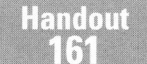
8a Two-part commands/questions

Touch the pen and spoon.

Touch the glass and comb.

Do dogs fly?

Is water wet?

8b Left/right discrimination

Touch your left cheek.

Touch your right knee.

Touch your right ear.

Touch your left elbow.

Initial Language Screen: Reading discrimination

9   Three-part commands/questions

Touch the spoon before the glass.

Touch the pen, tissue and comb.

Do mice have long tails?

Do teachers work in banks?

Initial Language Screen: Reading Discrimination

10 Four-part commands/questions

Touch the pen and comb after the spoon.

Is a kitten bigger than a fully grown cat?

Do fish and dogs both live in the sea?

Do you buy pills and deodorant in a chemist?

Initial Language Screen: Written Expression

1 Copying letters

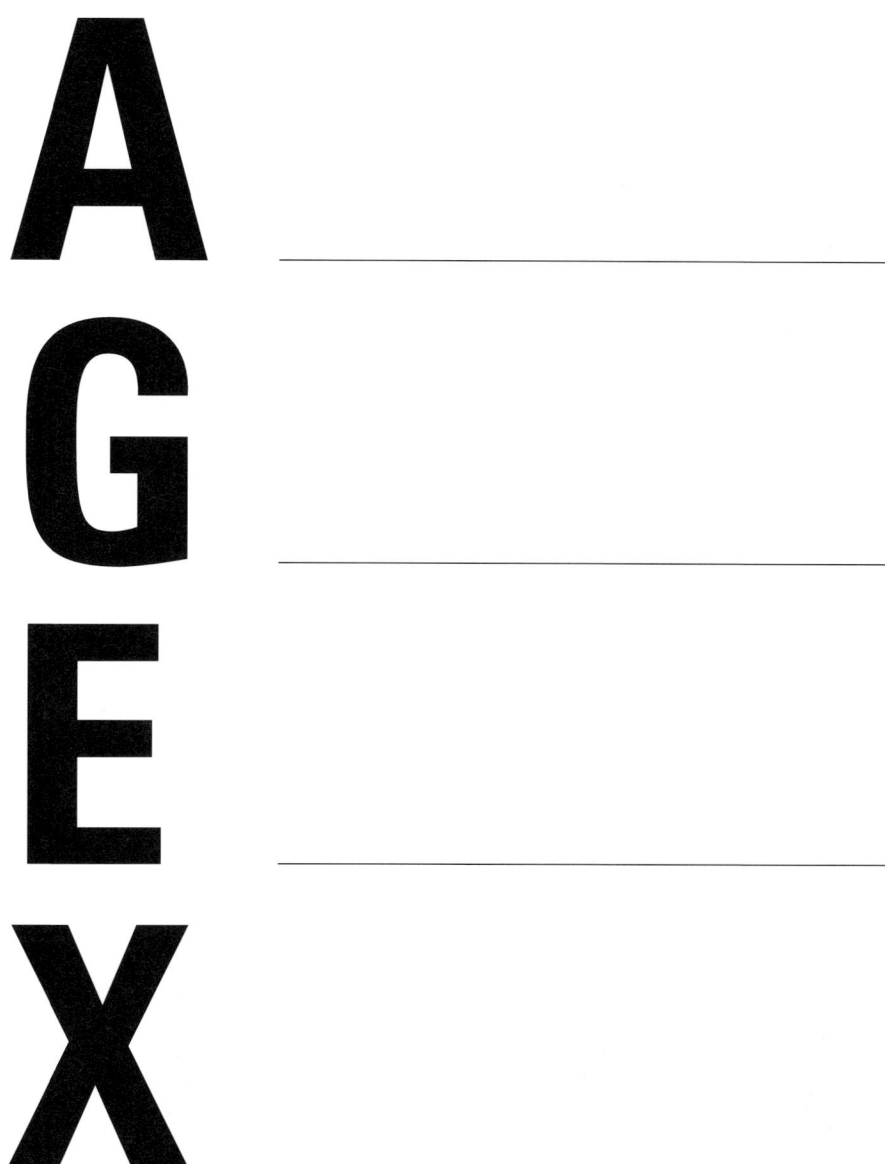

A _____

G _____

E _____

X _____

Recall

D J Y H

Initial Language Screen: Written Expression

2 Copying numbers

4 _____

12 _____

6 _____

34 _____

Recall

5 10 7 8

Handout
167
© F Sugden-Best 2002

3 Copying words

dog _____

back _____

drummer _____

wardrobe _____

Recall

box   **help**

rain   **pillow**

Initial Language Screen: Written Expression

7 Sentence completion

A loaf of _____ .

Children enjoy going to the _____ .

People go to the cinema to watch a _____ .

When it is cold you _____ the door.

Initial Language Screen: Written Expression

8a Sentence construction

house	**cat**
children	**food**
work	**late**

8b Sentence construction

Summertime	**barbeque**
garden	**Winter**
early	**lights**

Screen of Linguistic Concepts

Name _____ Date _____

QUESTIONS	SCORES
Inclusion/Exclusion (not, except, all, all but one, either)	
1 Point at a heart which is not red.	Y N NR
2 Point at either a blue or red heart.	Y N NR
3 Point at all the hearts except the yellow one.	Y N NR
4 Point at all but one heart.	Y N NR
TOTALS	
Temporal (after, before)	
5 Point at the blue oval before the green oval.	Y N NR
6 Point at the yellow oval after the red oval.	Y N NR
7 After pointing at the red oval, point at the green oval.	Y N NR
8 Before pointing at the blue oval, point at the yellow oval.	Y N NR
TOTALS	
Conditional (instead of, if, until, when)	
9 Point at the blue arrow instead of the yellow arrow.	Y N NR
10 Point at the red arrow if you see a green arrow.	Y N NR
11 Do not point at the blue arrow until I say 'now'.	Y N NR
12 When I have pointed at the red arrow, point at the green arrow.	Y N NR
TOTALS	
Coordination (and)	
13 Point at the blue and red crosses.	Y N NR
14 Point at the red and green crosses.	Y N NR
15 Point at the yellow and green crosses.	Y N NR
16 Point at the blue, yellow and red crosses.	Y N NR
TOTALS	
Quantitative (all, some, any one, all but one, first)	
17 Point at any one rectangle.	Y N NR
18 Point at all the rectangles, but the yellow one first.	Y N NR
19 Point at some of the rectangles.	Y N NR
20 Point at all but one of the rectangles.	Y N NR
TOTALS	

RESULTS/TOTAL CORRECT					
Inclusion/Exclusion	/4	**Temporal**	/4	**Conditional**	/4
Co-ordination	/4	**Quantitative**	/4		
			Total		**/20**

Screen of Linguistic Concepts (Inclusion/Exclusion)

P

This page may be photocopied
for instructional use only.
*Sourcebook for Assessing &
Maintaining Communication*
© F Sugden-Best 2002

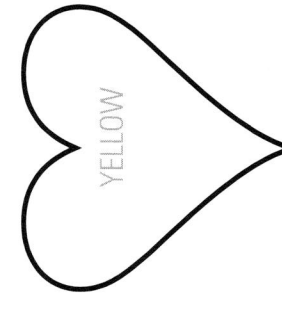

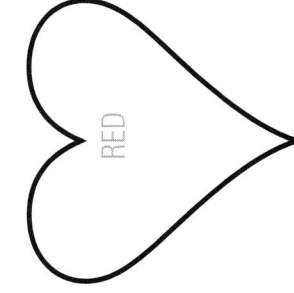

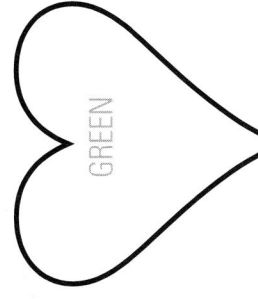

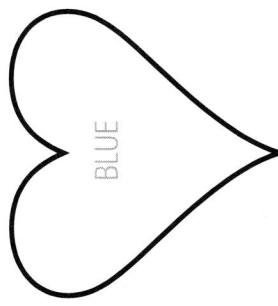

Screen of Linguistic Concepts (Temporal)

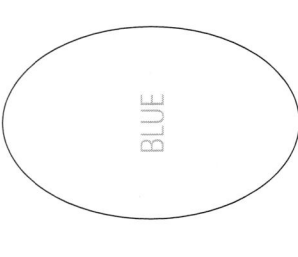

BLUE

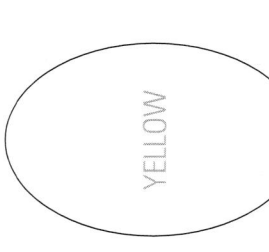

YELLOW

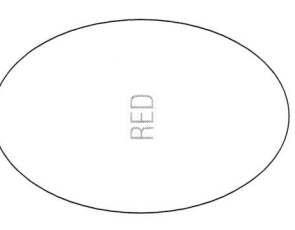

RED

GREEN

Screen of Linguistic Concepts (Conditional)

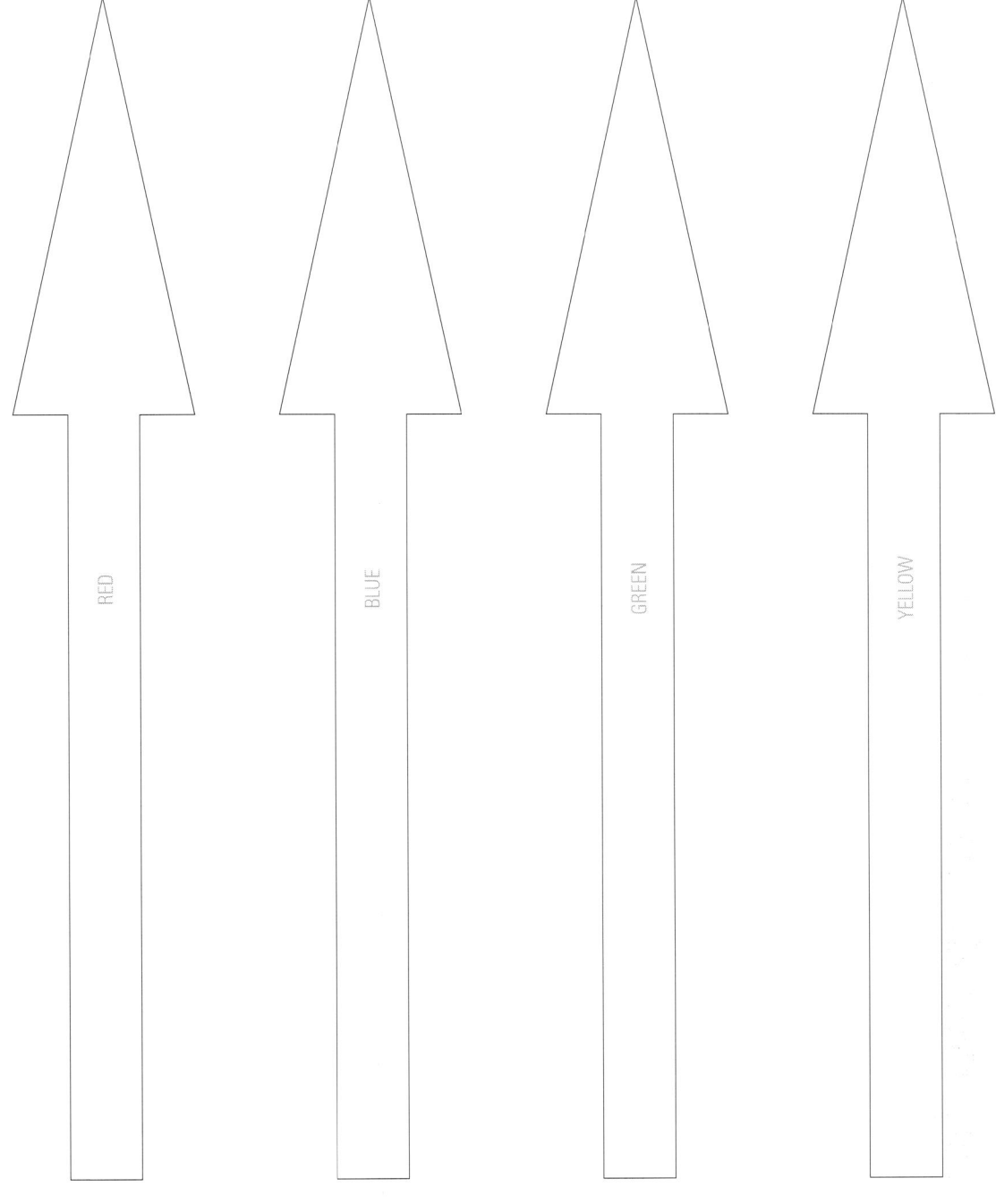

RED

BLUE

GREEN

YELLOW

Screen of Linguistic Concepts(Coordination)

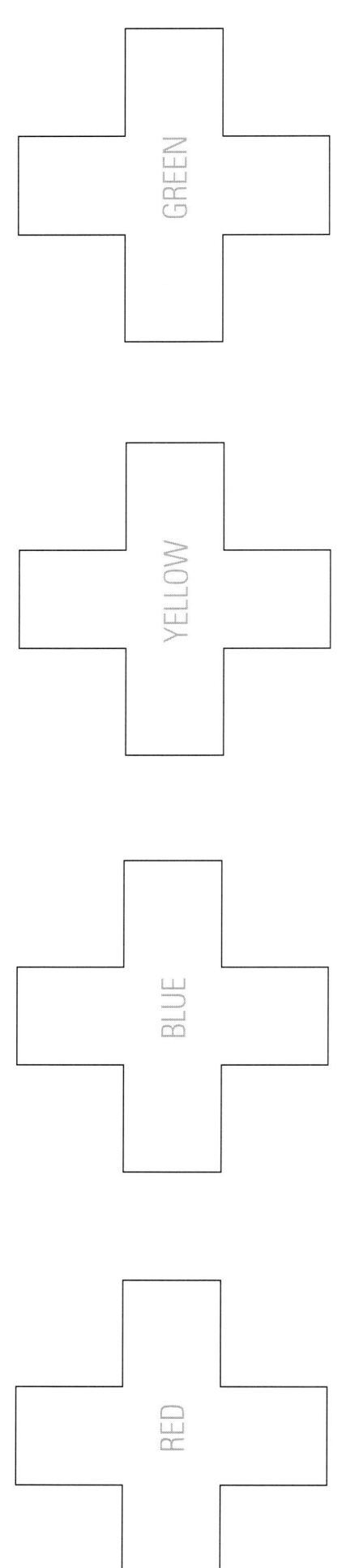

GREEN

YELLOW

BLUE

RED

Screen of Linguistic Concepts (Quantitative)

RED

BLUE

GREEN

YELLOW

Is It Dysphasia or Dementia?

Name _____ Date _____

COMMUNICATION

	DYSPHASIA	DEMENTIA
Gesture/Situation cues	Aids understanding	Cues may distract
Spoken/Written comprehension	Same level	Written worse
Peripheral sensory deficits	Can be compensated for	Affects performance adversely
Conversational sensitivity	Present	Reduced
Manner/type of presentation	May affect performance	Has greater effect
Immediate recall/ delayed recall	Both similar level	Immediate better than delayed
Expressive syntactic breakdown	Evident	Semantic rather than syntactic
Naming	Poor due to retrieval problems	Less affected, due to recognition problems
Phonological errors	More likely	Rare
Repetition high/low probability sentences	Equal difficulty	Low probability worse
Semantic/phonological cueing	Responds to cueing	Little response to cueing
Speech	Usually conveys/attempts to convey meaning	Empty speech/limited attempt to convey meaning
Automatic speech sequences	Does not always manage	Manages
Breakdown pattern	Evident, primarily due to auditory/visual problems	Less consistent
Gesture	May accompany speech	Rarely used

Is It Dysphasia or Dementia? *...continued*

GENERAL

	DYSPHASIA	DEMENTIA
Social behaviour	Appropriate	Inappropriate
Orientation in time and space	Good	Poor
Short-term memory	Good	Poor
Affect	Normal/Appropriate	Inappropriate, absent/ bizarre emotional responses
Personality	Intact	Changes
Activity	Purposeful (communication/ behaviour)	Purposeless (eg, talking to oneself)
Insight	Present, resulting in frustration	Little/limited, so frustration limited
Behaviour	Consistent	Inconsistent
Initiation	Does	Rarely does
Retain information and learn	Able to	Unable to

SCORES

	DYSPHASIA	DEMENTIA
Communication	/15	/15
General	/10	/10
TOTAL	**/25**	**/25**

Chapter 6

Augmentative and Alternative Communication Aids

This chapter contains:

1 **An alternative and augmentative communication screening form.** This includes sheets to assess tracking ability. These sheets can either be copied on to blank paper, or put on to acetates. The client has to trace the directions of arrows; look at numbers, letters and pictures, and pick the odd one out.

2 **Alphabet charts.** A selection of alphabet charts in a variety of layouts are included for direct access. In the Appendixes are examples of charts with a different colour on each line or every other line. The colour samples included in the Appendixes will give the clinician an indication of how effective the addition of colour can be. Blank charts can be photocopied and coloured to suit individual client needs. Word, phrase and picture charts have been omitted as it was felt that these would need to be designed by clinicians for individuals. Code lists would also fall into the same category. If certain items are not required on a chart – for example, end of word – these can be covered. The charts should be laminated or covered to prevent them from becoming dirty.

A basic alphabet chart can also be used in therapy with dysphasic or dysarthric clients – for example, by asking the client to find the correct letter prior to writing spontaneously; by then using the initial letter as a cue to say a word, or by encouraging the client to point to the first letter of each word as it is said in an attempt to slow down the speech – for example, of a client with Parkinson's disease.

3 **An elecotrnic communication aid caresheet.** This will be of value to nursing staff or anyone responsible for looking after electronic communication aids.

AAC Screening Form

Name _____ Date _____ _____

DOB _____ First language _____

Diagnosis _____

Date of onset _____

Have you tried a communication aid in the past?   YES/NO

If yes, what aid and what were the difficulties? _____

_____

Who do you regularly   Family ☐ Nurses ☐ Carers ☐ Friends ☐
communicate with?   Work colleagues ☐ Other _____

Current communication method _____

What are the problems with the current communication method? _____

_____

Will you have a wheelchair in the future?   YES/NO/POSSIBLY

In which settings will the   Home ☐ Work ☐ Further Education ☐
communication aid be used?   Other _____

Positioning/maximum time   Bed ____ mins   Chair ____ mins
tolerated   Wheelchair ___ mins

SENSORY FUNCTION

Visual	*(acuity, colour blindness, visual perception)*
Auditory	*(hearing aids)*
Tactile	*(reduced sensation)*

AAC Screening Form *...continued*

PSYCHOLOGICAL STATUS

Emotional status	*(lability)*
Insight	
Motivation	

PERCEPTUAL FUNCTION

Ability to trace *(Insert ticks and crosses to indicate ability, with comments if appropriate.)*	Horizontal left to right		
	Horizontal right to left		
	Top to bottom		
	Bottom to top		
	Diagonal bottom to top/right to left		
	Diagonal top to bottom/right to left		
	Diagonal bottom to top/left to right		
	Diagonal top to bottom/left to right		
	Point to four diamonds		
	Odd one out tasks	3 objects	4 objects
	Find letters A D U Z		
	Odd letter out	4 letters	5 letters
	Find letters A D F		
	Find numbers 4 8		
Ability to focus on an object	Consider size, colour, visual field		

AAC Screening Form   *...continued*

SPEECH AND LANGUAGE FUNCTION

Pre-morbid literacy skills	*(dyslexia, educational level/school/university)*
Speech and language diagnosis	Dysphasia Dysphonia Dysarthria Other _____
Pre-linguistic ability	Able to match objects YES/NO Able to match pictures YES/NO
Non-verbal expression	Facial expression Gesture/sign Eye gaze Other _____ Mouthing
Current literacy skills	Spelling Poor Average Excellent Reading Poor Average Excellent
Verbal comprehension ability	
Communication difficulties	
Level of pragmatic skills?	

COGNITIVE FUNCTION

Concentration/ Attention span	Concentration Poor Average Good Attention span < 10 mins > 10 mins < 20 mins > 20 mins
Memory deficits/ Learning potential	
Reasoning ability	
Initiation	
Orientation	Place Time Person
Ability to problem-solve	

AAC Screening Form   *...continued*

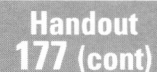

INITIAL COMMUNICATION AID TRIALLED

Aid trialled		
Access method		
Successful	YES	NO Reasons _____ _____ _____

SECONDARY COMMUNICATION AID TRIALLED

Aid trialled		
Access method		
Successful	YES	NO Reasons _____ _____ _____

Track from Left to Right

P

Track from Right to Left

Track from Top to Bottom

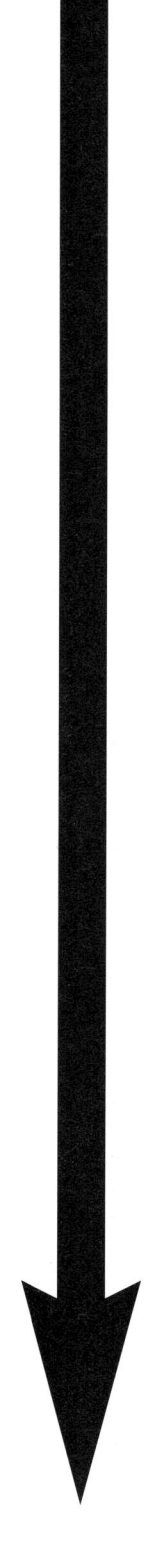

Track from Bottom to Top

Handout
181
Maintaining Communication

Track Diagonally Bottom to Top/Left to Right

Track Diagonally Top to Bottom/Left to Right

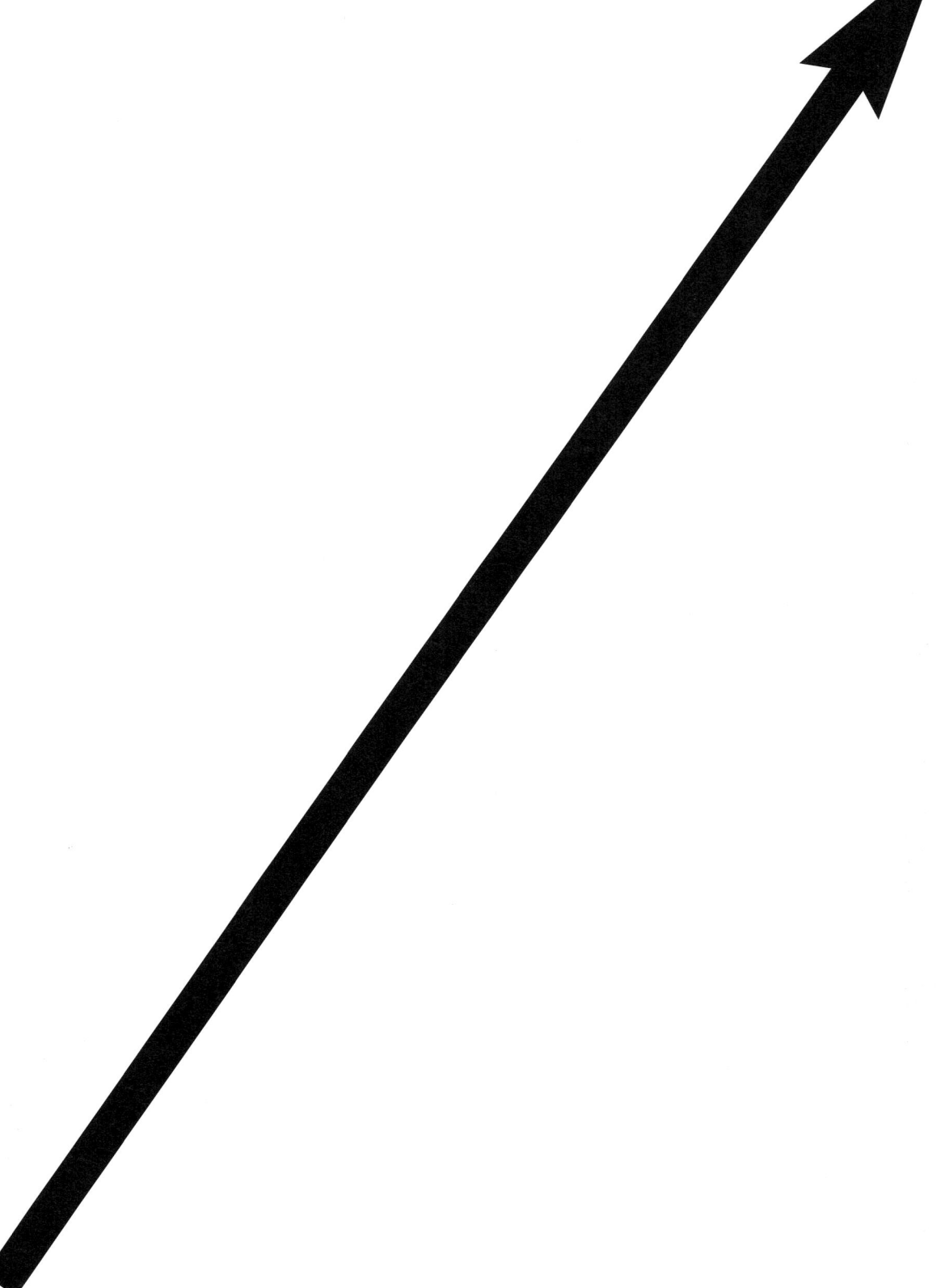

P

Track Diagonally Bottom to Top/Right to Left

Track Diagonally Top to Bottom/Right to Left

Point to the Four Diamonds

Find the Odd One Out

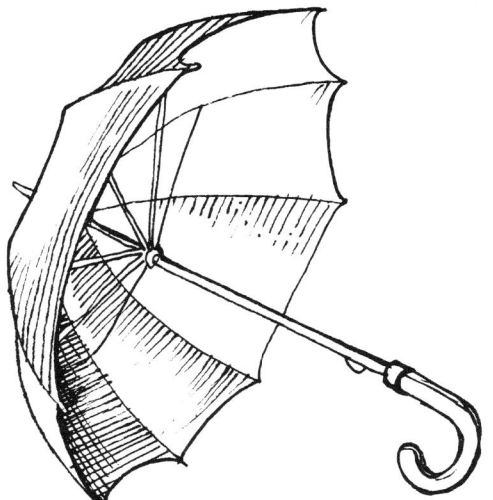

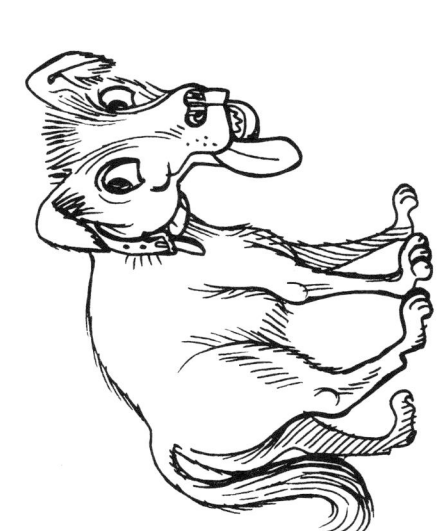

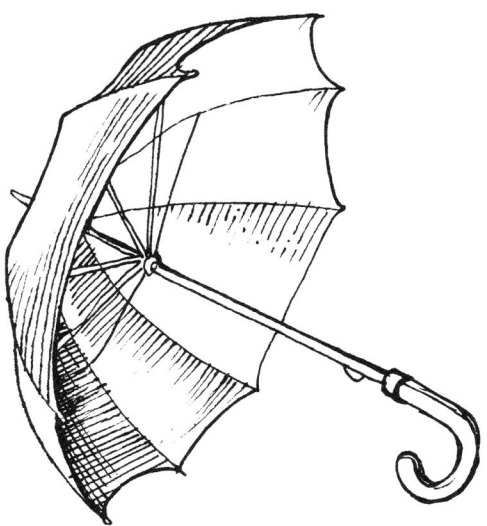

Find the Odd One Out

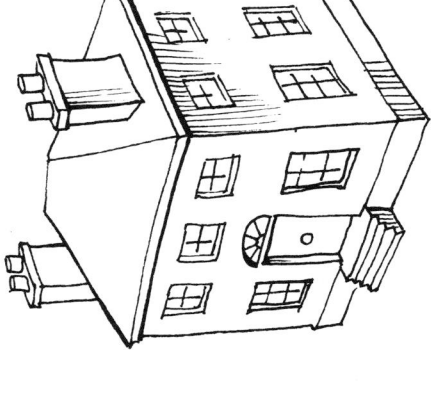

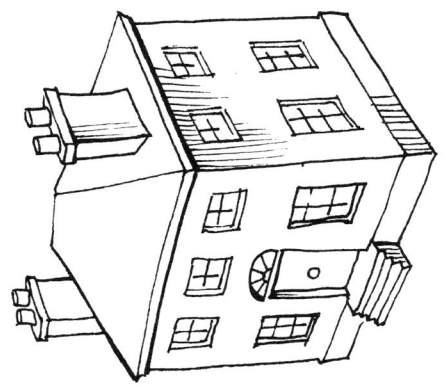

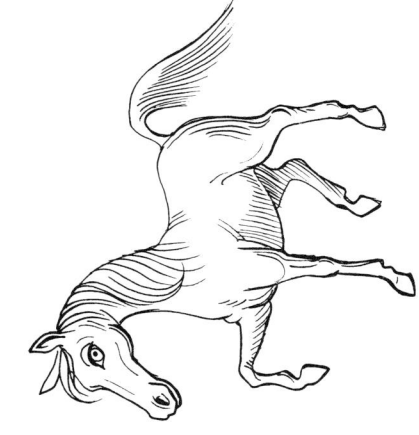

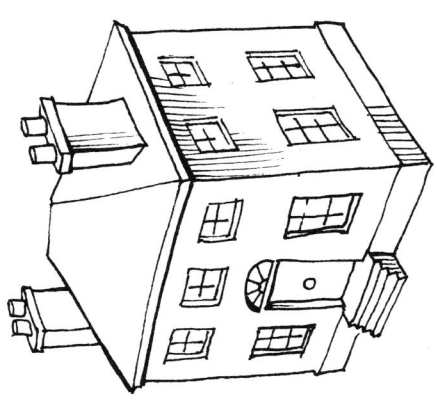

Find the Letters

D

N

A

U

Find the Odd One Out

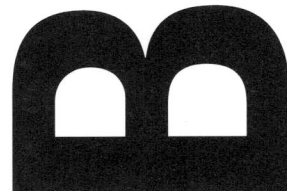

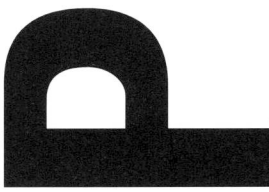

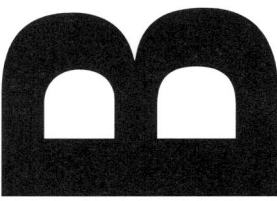

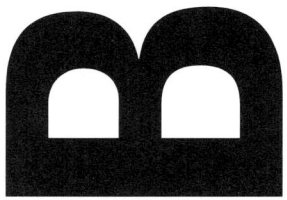

Find the Odd One Out

Find the Letters A, D and F

A B C D E F

Find the Numbers

8

9

1

4

Basic Alphabet Chart

Name _____

A	B	C	D	E	F	G
H	I	J	K	L	M	N
O	P	Q	R	S	T	U
V	W	X	Y	Z	9	8
1	2	3	4	5	6	7

LISTENER SCANNING

1 Go down – ie, A, H, O, V, 1.

2 Then go across – eg, V, W, X, Y, Z, 9, 8.

3 Write down the letters as you go along.

Basic Alphabet Chart (Black)

Name _____

A	B	C	D	E	F	G
H	I	J	K	L	M	N
O	P	Q	R	S	T	U
V	W	X	Y	Z	9	8
1	2	3	4	5	6	7

LISTENER SCANNING

1 Go down – ie, A, H, O, V, 1.

2 Then go across – eg, V, W, X, Y, Z, 9, 8.

3 Write down the letters as you go along.

Alphabet Chart with Code

Name _____

A	B	C	D	PLEASE
E	F	G	H	THANK YOU
			END OF WORD	CODE
I	J	K	L	M	N
O	P	Q	R	S	T
U	V	W	X	Y	Z

LISTENER SCANNING

1 Go down – ie, A, E, I, O, U.
2 Go across – eg, U, V, W, X, Y, Z.
3 Write down the letters as you go along.

Alphabet Chart with Code (Black)

Name ______________________

Handout 197

A	B	C	D	END OF WORD	PLEASE
E	F	G	H	CODE	THANK YOU
I	J	K	L	M	N
O	P	Q	R	S	T
U	V	W	X	Y	Z

LISTENER SCANNING

1 Go down – ie, A, E, I, O, U.

2 Go across – eg, U, V, W, X, Y, Z.

3 Write down the letters as you go along.

P

Alphabet Chart with Code and Numbers   Name _____

A	B	C	D	END OF WORD / CODE	1	6
E	F	G	H	PLEASE / THANK YOU	2	7
I	J	K	L	M	N	3	8
O	P	Q	R	S	T	4	9
U	V	W	X	Y	Z	5	0

LISTENER SCANNING

1 Go down – ie, A, E, I, O, U.
2 Then go across – eg, U, V, W, X, Y, Z, 5, 0.
3 Write down the letters as you go along.

*Sourcebook for Assessing &
Maintaining Communication*
© F Sugden-Best 2002

Alphabet Chart with Code and Numbers (Black)

Name _____

A	B	C	D	END OF WORD	CODE	1	6
E	F	G	H	PLEASE	THANK YOU	2	7
I	J	K	L	M	N	3	8
O	P	Q	R	S	T	4	9
U	V	W	X	Y	Z	5	0

LISTENER SCANNING

1 Go down – ie, A, E, I, O, U.

2 Then go across – eg, U, V, W, X, Y, Z, 5, 0.

3 Write down the letters as you go along.

1 2 3 4 5 6 7 8 9 0

Q W E R T Y U I O P

A S D F G H J K L

Z X C V B N M ?

SPACE

Alternative Keyboard Option

Name _____

A B C D

E F G H

I J K L

M N O P

Q R S T U

V W X Y Z

1 2 3 4 5

6 7 8 9 0

Guidelines for the Care of Electronic Communication Aids

1 Ensure the communication aid is kept well charged. Overnight charging is usually best.

Failure to charge regularly can result in the aid operating less efficiently, as it may run out of power during the day, or lose all its memory capacity, necessitating reprogramming.

2 When the communication aid is not being charged, remove the charger from the mains.

Chargers that are plugged in are a fire risk, like all electrical appliances. For this reason, aids should be charged where problems can be identified quickly, such as near a smoke detector.

3 Please keep the communication aid clean.

4 Remove the communication aid from the user's eating and drinking area to avoid any accidental spillages on to the aid.

5 Please report any breakdown, regardless of how minor it might seem, to the speech and language therapist as soon as possible.
Contact number _____.

Appendixes

These appendixes include:

Samples of colour sheets. These are for information purposes to illustrate how some of the sheets and charts look when colour is added.

Appendix 1
Pitch Diagrams

Name _____ Date _____

1 Crescendo

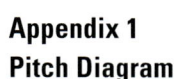

2 Diminuendo

Appendix 1
Pitch Diagrams

Name _____ Date _____

3 Crescendo/Diminuendo

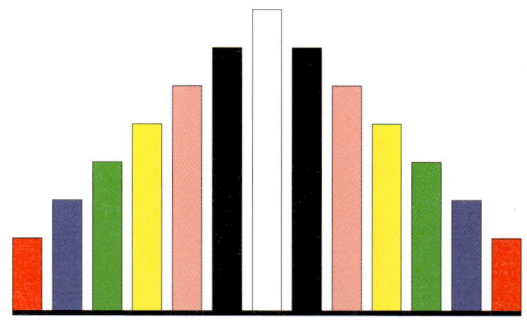

4 Diminuendo/Crescendo

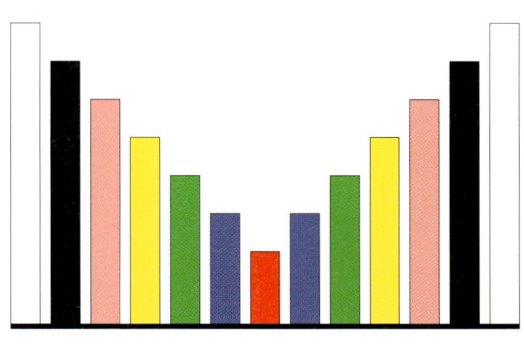

Appendix 1
Pitch Diagrams

Name _____ Date _____

5 Pitch jumps

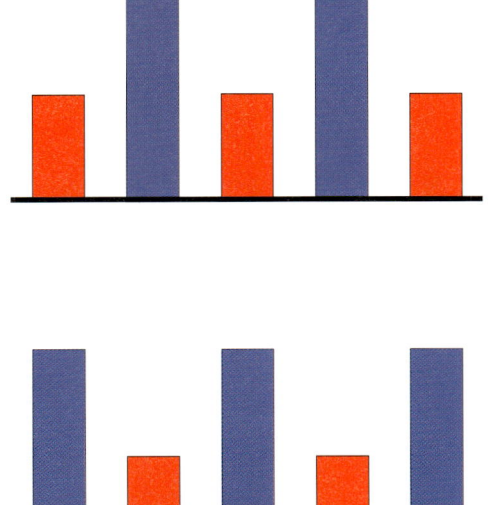

Appendix 2
Initial Language Screen: Visual Matching
1 – Colour to Colour

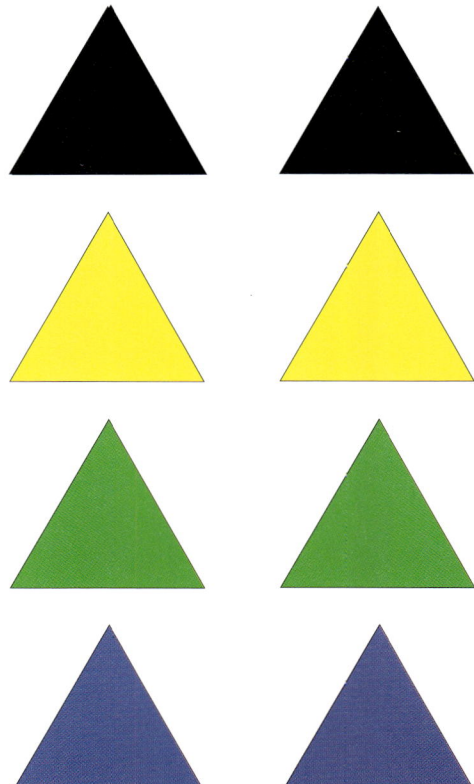

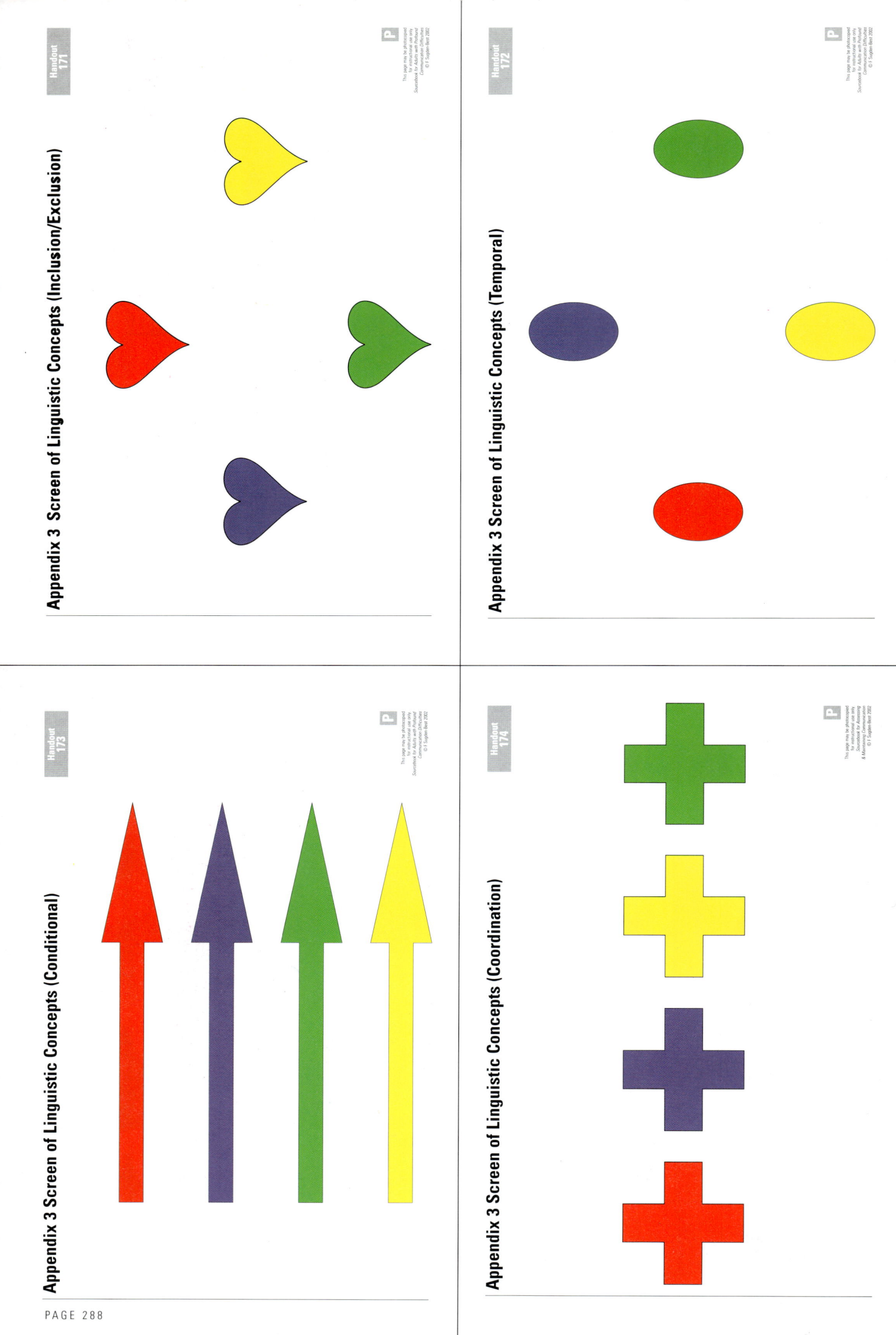

Appendix 3 Screen of Linguistic Concepts (Inclusion/Exclusion)

Appendix 3 Screen of Linguistic Concepts (Temporal)

Appendix 3 Screen of Linguistic Concepts (Conditional)

Appendix 3 Screen of Linguistic Concepts (Coordination)

Appendix 3 Screen of Linguistic Concepts (Quantitative)

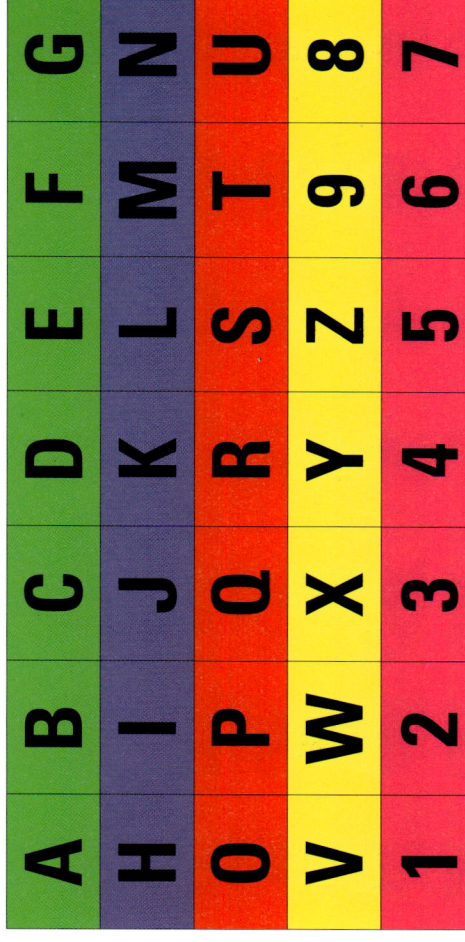

Appendix 4 Basic alphabet chart (A, H, O, V) – 5 colours

A	B	C	D	E	F	G
H	I	J	K	L	M	N
O	P	Q	R	S	T	U
V	W	X	Y	Z	9	8
1	2	3	4	5	6	7

LISTENER SCANNING
1 Go down – ie, A, H, O, V, 1.
2 Then go across – eg. V, W, X, Y, Z, 9, 8.
3 Write down the letters as you go along.

Appendix 4 Basic alphabet chart (A, H, O, V) – alternating colour

A	B	C	D	E	F	G
H	I	J	K	L	M	N
O	P	Q	R	S	T	U
V	W	X	Y	Z	9	8
1	2	3	4	5	6	7

LISTENER SCANNING
1 Go down – ie, A, H, O, V, 1.
2 Then go across – eg. V, W, X, Y, Z, 9, 8.
3 Write down the letters as you go along.

Appendix 4 Alphabet chart (A, E, I, O, U) – 5 colours

A	B	C	D	END OF WORD	PLEASE
E	F	G	H	CODE	THANK YOU
I	J	K	L	M	N
O	P	Q	R	S	T
U	V	W	X	Y	Z

LISTENER SCANNING
1 Go down – ie, A, E, I, O, U.
2 Go across – eg, U, V, W, X, Y, Z.
3 Write down the letters as you go along.

Handout 198

Appendix 4 Alphabet chart (A, E, I, O, U) with numbers – alternating colours

A	B	C	D	END OF WORD	CODE	1	6
E	F	G	H	PLEASE	THANK YOU	2	7
I	J	K	L	M	N	3	8
O	P	Q	R	S	T	4	9
U	V	W	X	Y	Z	5	0

LISTENER SCANNING
1. Go down – ie, A, E, I, O, U.
2. Then go across – eg, U, V, W, X, Y, Z, 5, 0.
3. Write down the letters as you go along.

Handout 199

Appendix 4 Black alphabet chart (A, E, I, O, U) with numbers – 5 colours

A	B	C	D	END OF WORD	CODE	1	6
E	F	G	H	PLEASE	THANK YOU	2	7
I	J	K	L	M	N	3	8
O	P	Q	R	S	T	4	9
U	V	W	X	Y	Z	5	0

LISTENER SCANNING
1. Go down – ie, A, E, I, O, U.
2. Then go across – eg, U, V, W, X, Y, Z, 5, 0.
3. Write down the letters as you go along.

Handout 195

Appendix 4 Basic alphabet chart (A, H, O, V) – 5 colours

A	B	C	D	E	F	G
H	I	J	K	L	M	N
O	P	Q	R	S	T	U
V	W	X	Y	Z	9	8
1	2	3	4	5	6	7

LISTENER SCANNING
1. Go down – ie, A, H, O, V, 1.
2. Then go across – eg, V, W, X, Y, Z, 9, 8.
3. Write down the letters as you go along.

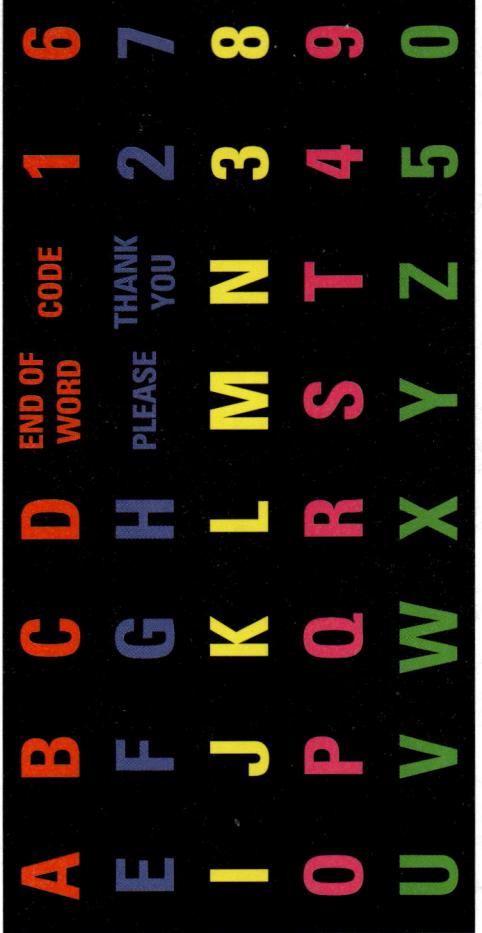